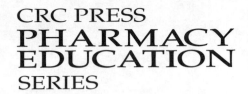

CRC PRESS PHARMACY EDUCATION SERIES

PHARMACEUTICAL CARE:
INSIGHTS *from* COMMUNITY PHARMACISTS

PHARMACEUTICAL CARE:
INSIGHTS *from* COMMUNITY PHARMACISTS

WILLIAM N. TINDALL
MARSHA K. MILLONIG

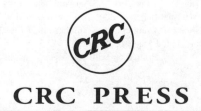

CRC PRESS

Boca Raton   London   New York   Washington, D.C.

Library of Congress Cataloging-in-Publication Data

Pharmaceutical care: insights from community pharmacists / William N. Tindall and
Marsha K. Millonig.
     p. ; cm.— (CRC pharmacy education series)
Includes bibliographical references.
ISBN 1-56676-953-1
    1. Pharmacy—Practice. 2. Pharmacists—Interviews. I. Tindall, William N. II. Millonig,
Marsha K. III. Series.
    [DNLM: 1. Pharmaceutical Services. 2. Pharmacy. QV 737 P5344 2002]
RS100 .P437 2002
615'.1'068—dc21

2002073642
CIP

Visit the CRC Press Web site at www.crcpress.com

© 2003 by CRC Press LLC

No claim to original U.S. Government works
International Standard Book Number 1-56676-953-1
Library of Congress Card Number 2002073642
Printed in the United States of America 1 2 3 4 5 6 7 8 9 0
Printed on acid-free paper

DEDICATION

To Bruce A. Siecker for his loyal friendship,
Joseph A. Oddis for his gentle wisdom,
in Bill's family: Sylvia, Christine,
Laura and Michael,
and in Marsha's family: Lawrence, Mary,
Trisha, Michael, Adam, and Aaron
who all supported us with uncommon love
so we could reach our dreams

PREFACE

A widely accepted definition for *pharmaceutical care* as found in the American Society of Health-System Pharmacists' (ASHP's) Residency Manual is "the responsible provision of drug therapy for the purpose of achieving specific outcomes that improve a patient's quality of life." However, a more easily understood definition was approved during the 1989 Pharmacy in the 21st Century (P21) Conference. That definition uses plain language to convey what contemporary pharmacy practice is all about, i.e., helping people make the best use of their medications. Speaking and writing about this definition, which has become the mission statement for pharmacy practice, ASHP Executive Vice President William A. Zellmer states:

> Let me emphasize again the key role of the staff planning committee for the 1989 P21 conference. These individuals were pharmacists responsible for the practice development programs of the national pharmacist organizations. They labored over putting together an influential program and exceeded their expectations. They worked together well and were able to focus on advancement of the profession while transcending the sometimes narrow-minded self-interests of individual organizations that have been known to spoil similar attempts at collaborative work. They served as vectors, carrying the infectious enthusiasm from the P21 program into their separate organizations. It is because of their efforts that the outer reaches of pharmacy in the United States began to hear about pharmaceutical care shortly after October 1989, and those conversations are still going on today.*

---

* Zellmer, W.A., *Role of Pharmacy Organizations in Transforming the Profession*, American Pharmaceutical Association Annual Meeting, March 2001, San Francisco, CA. Members of the P21 planning committee include William N. Tindall (NCPA), chairman; Maude A. Babington (ASCP); Marsha K. Millonig (NACDS); Richard P. Penna (AACP); Dorothy A. Wade (National Pharmaceutical Council); C. Edwin Webb (APhA); and William A. Zellmer (ASHP).

The P21 mission for pharmacy practice provides the basis for this text. We believe it not our task to make a case for the mission. Others have done that and done it very well. Our text was written with one simple goal in mind — to bring its readers insights from a few pharmacists who are part of a professional vanguard. These professionals are innovative. They practice with pride and are committed to deliver on a professional covenant and to conduct the practice of pharmacy to the best of their abilities.

Our interviews were conducted with pharmacists who do not see themselves as leaders or innovators, but were willing to provide lessons worth sharing. They are community pharmacists who practice in professionally satisfying ways that may not match an academic or textbook definition of pharmaceutical care, but they are the unsung practitioners and some of the first to make the practice of pharmaceutical care visible in community settings. Since 1996 the authors interviewed more than 50 pharmacists in different practice settings. Those chosen for this book are pharmacists who were among the first to develop these patient focused services. Some of them have never been featured in an article or book on pharmaceutical care. They stand out from their peers in that they led change in the particular practice setting in which they were working. They are committed to providing patient care and are willing to expend considerable personal time and energy to achieve this goal. They are different from their peers in their passion for practice and their resulting achievements.

The *Oxford American Dictionary* defines an innovator as "one who introduces a new process or way of doing things." While these practitioners do not always apply that label to themselves, they are innovators from our point of view. We hope their stories show the contrast in their career paths to other pharmacists who practice in a more traditional dispensing model.

When we interviewed our community pharmacists we wanted to find out:

■ What makes them stand out from their peers?
■ What makes them fight for their goals and ambitions?
■ Why do they think hard work and perseverance are stronger contributors to their success than a high grade-point average in college or a genetically determined high intellect?
■ What value systems were in play and contributed to the pharmacist's professional success?

Thus, we talked to some special pharmacists about their:

- Integrity
- Self-control
- Family, friends, peers
- Mentors and college experiences
- Ability to get along with people, trade-off between their focus on helping people vs. gaining commercial success
- Influence of professional commitment on lifestyles

From our background readings and work with practitioners to date we created a standard interview guide, a copy of which may be found in Appendix A.

This book is about lessons learned from courageous innovators who sought a better and more satisfying professional life. They did so by walking a pathway guided by faith and a conviction that doing so was important to them. They were also guided by a mission that securing a high level of professional satisfaction could be reached by delivering the best service they could, believing in the covenant between pharmacist and patient, and accepting the challenge to redefine and revitalize themselves.

Pharmacy is the nation's third largest health profession. Today there are almost 195,000 licensed pharmacists in the U.S., 120,000 practicing in community pharmacies, according to 2001 data from the Bureau of Health Professionals. This is where these authors looked for pharmacist heroes to interview for this book because this is where pharmaceutical care is judged, accepted, and ultimately purchased. These are also the venues where pharmacists need the most help and the tools to survive in turbulent, changing markets. These practices have mixed support from consumers and less support from a health care system that offers little in the way of help and resources that would pay for a pharmacist's cognitive skills and services.

For 30 years, a Harris survey reports pharmacists as America's most trusted professionals. This distinction is a well-earned compliment. Recently, and after considerable professional effort, pharmacists are also being recognized for their direct participation in patient medication management as discriminating resources of information and as counselors on behaviors that benefit patients. Pharmacists can also be proud that the World Health Organization (WHO) has praised their importance as communicators and caregivers.* The WHO further describes pharmacists as having the skills and opportunities to improve treatment and quality of life outcomes for many.

Making a difference is what this book is all about. We trust it will be used as a motivational resource providing help to pharmacists wanting to adopt expanded caregiver and communicator roles. The fact you are reading it means you are interested in making a difference also.

Bill Tindall
School of Medicine
Wright State University
Dayton, OH

Marsha Millonig
Catalyst Enterprises, LLC
Eagan, MN

---

* Zellmer, W.A., *Role of Pharmacy Organizations in Transforming the Profession*, APhA Annual Meeting, March 2001, San Francisco, CA.

THE AUTHORS

William N. Tindall, Ph.D., R.Ph., C.A.E., is currently a professor of family medicine research and director of the Alliance for Research in Community Health at the School of Medicine's Department of Family Medicine at Wright State University, Dayton, Ohio. He assists in a team approach to community-based, collaborative and participatory research activities. Previously he was executive director of the American College of Managed Care Medicine (ACMCM). Prior to joining the ACMCM, Dr. Tindall served as the first executive director of the Academy of Managed Care Pharmacy (AMCP) in Washington, D.C. He helped build AMCP into a national voice for managed care pharmacy, served as a registered lobbyist on managed care issues, and launched the *Journal of Managed Care Pharmacy*. Dr. Tindall also served 8 years as the first vice president of professional affairs for the National Community Pharmacist Association (NCPA).

Before moving to Washington, D.C., Dr. Tindall served 10 years as a faculty member, department chair, and associate dean at Creighton University College of Pharmacy. He has also held teaching appointments at Ferris State College in Michigan, the University of Rhode Island, and the University of Saskatchewan.

Dr. Tindall earned his B.S. in pharmacy from the University of Saskatchewan, his M.S. in administration from Long Island University, and his Ph.D. in pharmaceutical economics from the University of Pittsburgh. He completed postdoctoral training at the University of Southern California School of Medicine, and earned his certified association executive (C.A.E.) designation from the American Society of Association Executives.

In 1996, Dr. Tindall was recognized by *Drug Store News* as one of America's most influential pharmacists. He has co-authored two books on pharmacy practice and communication skills (see Tindall, W.N., Beardsley, R.A., and Kimberlin, C.A., *Communication Skills for Pharmacy Practice,* Lippincott, Williams, & Wilkins, Baltimore, MD, 2000, now in its fourth edition; and *A Guide to Managed Care Medicine*, Aspen Publishers, Gaithersburg, MD, 2000). He has also published a novel and more than 60 articles on pharmacy practice and managed care. Dr. Tindall has raised several million dollars by successfully obtaining funding for over 30 grants. He has written guest articles on pharmacoeconomics for *Business and Health*. Dr. Tindall has given more than 200 presentations to national and international audiences on managed care, pharmacy practice, management, and communicating with patients.

Marsha Millonig, M.B.A., R.Ph., is the president of Catalyst Enterprises a health care consulting, writing and research firm in Eagan, MN. The company specializes in projects that help drive organizations and individuals among pharmacy, distribution, and manufacturing to become more efficient and value-added providers of health care in an effort to improve patient health outcomes. Prior to forming this firm, Ms. Millonig was vice president of research and information for the Healthcare Distribution Management Association (HDMA), formerly the National Wholesale Druggists' Association (NWDA). In this position, she led HDMA's research and intelligence efforts, which included the creation of an environmental-scanning and trend-tracking service, and related publications, including the popular *Industry Profile and Healthcare Factbook*. She also served as vice president of the HDMA Healthcare Foundation, the association's research and philanthropic arm.

Ms. Millonig has led a number of cutting-edge research projects in areas such as patient privacy and confidentiality of medical records, components of successful pharmaceutical care, biotechnology and its impact on health care, regulatory compliance costs, and other distribution-related work. She joined HDMA in 1991 spearheading the group's supply chain distribution, information, and e-commerce systems and standards efforts.

Before joining HDMA, Ms. Millonig spent nearly 8 years with the National Association of Chain Drug Stores (NACDS) working with chain pharmacy executives on issues in pharmacy operations, professional and state government affairs, and pharmacy education and practice. She was actively involved with the International Pharmaceutical Federation (FIP), and is currently a member of many pharmacy and professional associations.

Ms. Millonig is a registered pharmacist. She received her bachelor's degree from the University of Minnesota College of Pharmacy, completed a residency in association management with the American Society of Health-Systems Pharmacists (ASHP) in 1983, and earned an M.B.A., with a marketing and finance concentration, in 1988 from the University of Maryland College of Business and Management. She is also a practicing pharmacist, having volunteered at the Whitman Walker Elizabeth Taylor AIDS Clinic in Washington, D.C. from 1995–2002. Her knowledge of supply system issues, from manufacturing to distribution to pharmacy to patient care, is diverse, and she is often asked to share her expertise on evolving business models and the trends leading to their development.

CONTENTS

SECTION II: UNCOMMON PEOPLE

SECTION III: LESSONS LEARNED FROM PASSIONATE PHARMACISTS

I

COMMON PURPOSE

1

THE DREAM OF PHARMACEUTICAL CARE

I have a dream.

—Rev. Dr. Martin Luther King, Jr.

For me, heroes are ordinary people doing extraordinary things for the greater good.

—Tom Brokaw, NBC News, following the September 11, 2001 disaster

Health professionals are trusted individuals who provide health care services and products, consistently using the highest levels of professionalism demanded by their communities. Pharmacists personify this description and are well educated and disciplined in order to live up to their obligations. Whenever pharmacists resolve a patient's medication needs, research and answer a patient's questions about prescription or nonprescription medications, or go the extra mile to make sure a medication being used is appropriate, they become a living testament to the core values of their profession. They care for and advise clients, who, by trusting pharmacists, empower them to apply their professional judgment and creative problem-solving abilities. Pharmacists accept responsibility for their actions, often with little appreciation from those they helped.

That best portion of a good man's life; His little, nameless, unremembered acts of kindness and of love.

—William Wordsworth

3

In today's rich and diverse communities there is a call for professional medication management. Pharmacists are trained to provide this service, and do so with compassion and at a level of individualized patient care unmatched by any other health care profession. Recently there has been a movement to define and promote a level of pharmaceutical service excellence, documenting the education and contributions of pharmacists that qualify them as being more than simple retailers of medicine. This movement has been a part of the professional literature for more than two decades, and while it was first labeled "pharmaceutical care," it is also termed "comprehensive pharmacy services," "medication management," and "pharmacist care." Today it is more than encouraging pharmacists to take more responsibility. It has become a movement to help the public take more responsibility for their own health and to challenge pharmacists to help the public achieve better medication outcomes by working with them, their other caregivers, and physicians.

Pharmacists know it is a privilege to serve their communities as health professionals. They also know this privilege is bestowed by those who grant them their licenses — the public. But to improve the health of the public as a national goal, the pharmacy profession needs its wisest, most experienced, and charismatic leaders to organize the pharmaceutical care movement and rally public support. To accomplish this, innovative practitioners have to blaze a trail on which others can follow.

A good example of a trailblazer who forged a new pathway can be found in the work of Dr. Martin Luther King, Jr. in the civil rights movement. Dr. King did not stand on the steps of the Lincoln Memorial in Washington, D.C., and state that he was a leader with a defined mission statement and predetermined goals and objectives. Rather, he fueled the imagination of his audience when he shouted, "I have a dream...." That phrase galvanized those who understood that the pathway to a new national objective would be the result of how people could follow the roadmap he had prepared for them. Dr. King's motivating speech appealed to everyone's inner self or spiritual side by giving words to a complex and emotionally laden idea. It empowered people to realize they could have the same dream if they would act on their interpretation of his dream. He knew full well that we live in a diverse society where plurality is good for its health, but survival depends on policies that are fair and applied equitably to all within its borders.

This dream of pharmaceutical care, however, is one that will be only pretty words unless a few brave souls say, "Hey! I have a dream too," and "I can do a better job of caring for those who come to my pharmacy." There is no charismatic leader in pharmacy like Dr. King, but there are hundreds of innovative practitioners achieving their own dream of a better profession.

If we passionately believe in something and if we work hard at achieving our dreams, we will get exactly what we need exactly when we need it.

—Alan Hobson, mountaineer and Everest summiteer

There should be no job description for pharmaceutical care. However academics and professionals describe and define pharmaceutical care, some claiming it is the future of the profession. In reality, pharmaceutical care is more about a priority for delivering care that either some will adopt or adapt as local conditions, patient care settings, and economic or business parameters permit, or that some will never adopt or adapt unless regulatory forces legislate action. Pharmacy's professional societies, colleges, and many focused study groups have all agreed that it is the "basis of a bright future and the manifest mission of the profession."[1] College and academic resources are now educating students in pharmaceutical care precepts in both community pharmacy and institutional settings.[2]

In the mid-1990s, as part of an American Pharmaceutical Association (APhA) initiative to lobby the Clinton administration's health reform movement, a price tag was put on the nation's "other" drug problem. Researchers estimated that the annual cost of the morbidity and mortality associated with America's ambulatory population for prescription drugs was $76.6 billion, and that this sum matched nearly dollar for dollar what was spent by the same population to correct drug-related problems.[3] In a follow-up report, the same authors presented a model showing that 59.6% or nearly 60 cents of every dollar spent on drug-related problems could be avoided by community pharmacists' interventions.[4] An updated study published in 2001 raised the estimated drug morbidity and mortality cost to $177 billion annually.[5] In contrast, pharmaceutical care for patients with chronic health conditions appears to be associated with a modest increase in health care utilization, even without a cost-substitution effect. However, pharmaceutical care may offer the important benefit of assuring a more appropriate use of medications and a way for pharmacists to contribute to the monitoring of patients.[6] In an editorial, the authors propose a design model to evaluate community-based pharmaceutical care citing that as an innovative program it will need to be evaluated in terms of patient clinical outcomes, such as disease state, quality of life, and cost effectiveness.[7] Following on this premise, other researchers endorsed the idea but note that such innovations, given the increasing complexity of medication regimens, must include increased community pharmacist involvement while noting:

- Barriers to interventions will be considerable.
- Interventions will require partnerships.
- Interventions will need to be potent enough to effect change.
- Interventions will not be able to place too much responsibility on the pharmacist.
- Interventions cannot be economically cumbersome.[8]

But how does a community pharmacist "intervene" in a drug-related problem if he or she is to make a difference in both cost of care and quality of care? And, as one study comments, how can pharmacists maintain a commitment to provide medication interventions when it is reported they find an average of three drug-therapy problems per hundred patients?[9] It could be argued that the pharmaceutical care approach requires a preparedness to act on behalf of all patients while searching for that small 3%. It could also be argued that a pharmacist needs a systematic approach to make effective pharmaceutical care his or her practice modus operandi; the APhA has created a five-step process (Figure 1.1) to achieve this goal.[10] This five-step process is an ideal way to help pharmacists determine whether or not a patient's needs are being met. The most challenging

1. A professional relationship with the patient must be established.
2. Patient-specific medical information must be collected, organized, recorded, and maintained.
3. Patient-specific medical information must be evaluated and a drug-therapy plan developed mutually with the patient.
4. The pharmacist must ensure that the patient has all the supplies, knowledge, and information necessary to carry out the drug-therapy plan.
5. The pharmacist must review, monitor, and modify the therapeutic plan as necessary and appropriate in concert with the patient and health care team.

Figure 1.1 The American Pharmaceutical Association pharmaceutical care process.

aspect of this process, however, is getting that inner dream acted upon and finding the motivation to apply innovation to pharmaceutical care in real-world settings.

WHAT MOTIVATES A PHARMACIST TO EMBRACE PHARMACEUTICAL CARE?

Nothing happens unless first a dream.

—Carl Sandberg

In one research article it was demonstrated that pharmacists who are able to work collaboratively with patients have immediate, objective, point-of-care patient data, and possess the necessary knowledge, skills, and resources can provide an advanced level of care resulting in successful management of dislipidemia.[11] In the survey, pharmacists working in 26 pharmacies in 12 states intervened for 3 years providing dislipidemia treatment interventions to 397 patients. Each of the 26 pharmacies was selected because one of its pharmacists demonstrated a "readiness to provide basic pharmaceutical care." This readiness was assessed by each community pharmacist having the following resources:

- Semi-private area for counseling
- Technician support
- Documentation systems
- Experience with disease management programs
- Good interpersonal communication skills
- Ability to implement point-of-sale testing technology
- Willingness to undertake a $2\frac{1}{2}$-day training program

The results of this study revealed pharmacists could make a two- to fourfold improvement in patient adherence to a medication regimen as well as increase treatment goal objectives. This study did not examine the mind-set among study pharmacists or when and why they decided it was right for them to try a new professional paradigm.

Other similar studies in the professional literature show that meeting the challenges of pharmaceutical care is not restricted to the U.S. For example, in Denmark where a prospective, controlled, multicenter study of 500 asthma patients was administered, pharmacists managed a seven-step cyclical outcome improvement process that required cooperation among pharmacists, patients, and physicians. It was demonstrated that pharmacist monitoring was an effective strategy for improving the quality of drug therapy for asthma patients.[12] However, the study failed to address when, where, how, and why pharmacists shift into a pharmaceutical care practice mode. It also failed to reveal if such a shift caused professional angst and, if so, for what time period. Or did it start with the motivation to intervene in just one disease state? Or was it a general philosophical bent to intervene in all opportunities of therapy management?

Obviously, pharmaceutical care interventions cannot occur for every prescription brought into a community pharmacy or each medication order filled in a hospital or other institution. It is not feasible, nor is it necessary. For example, in one study by the American Society of Health System Pharmacists (ASHP), responding hospitals and health system institutions found the source of pharmaceutical care interventions as being:

- Physician orders (68%)
- Patient requests (57%)
- Discharge orders for targeted drugs (37%)
- Targeted food–drug interactions (27%)
- Targeted diseases (14%)
- Orders for drugs with drug–drug interactions (14%)[13]

Since documentation of pharmaceutical care interventions is a critical component of its definition and is its best hope for reimbursement or compensation, only 57% of the ASHP study institutions reported pharmacists as being required to document inpatient medication counseling. However, as pharmaceutical care becomes more common in community settings, pharmacists must independently undertake the risks of:

- Clinical monitoring
- Documenting interventions
- Documenting and evaluating outcomes
- Focusing on chronic care conditions such as asthma, hypertension, diabetes, obesity, arthritis, and dislipidemia[9]

In several chronic care situations the willingness to participate in community pharmaceutical care programs was documented as being motivated by opportunities to:

- Increase customer loyalty
- Increase job satisfaction
- Gain additional compensation[14]

Despite the particular motivation behind them, efforts to inform and encourage patients in the appropriate use of prescribed therapies have increased therapy adherence rates.

Whatever you can do, or dream you can do, begin it. Boldness has genius, power and magic in it.

—Goethe

HOW CAN PHARMACISTS DO MORE?

In 1997 the National Wholesale Druggists Association (NWDA), now called the Healthcare Distribution Management Association (HDMA), in partnership with the APhA released a much-anticipated, extensive, and eventually much-heralded planning resource. To help pharmacists deliver pharmaceutical care, the APhA–NWDA Concept Pharmacy resource consists of:

■ A two-part video, "Pharmaceutical Care in Action," and "A Road-Map to Patient-Focused Care"
■ An annotated bibliography of studies outlining the benefits of pharmaceuticals and comprehensive pharmaceutical services
■ *The Guidebook of Pharmaceutical Care Resources*, which lists sources of help with information systems, facility redesign, pharmaceutical care education on patient education, disease state management, patient monitoring
■ A pamphlet offering quotes from 17 pharmacists
■ A survey form to assess a pharmacist's readiness to deliver pharmaceutical care[15]

The survey to assess readiness to deliver pharmaceutical care is based on Prochaska's Model of Change.[16] Prochaska states that people move through five stages of change in order to adopt new behavior:

1. Precontemplation
2. Contemplation
3. Preparation
4. Action
5. Maintenance

Because the APhA–NWDA survey is a self-assessment tool, there has not been any literature that aggregates groups of pharmacists. Such an aggregate would provide insight into whatever relevance each of Prochaska's five stages may play in a pharmacist's move to pharmaceutical care. It might also reveal what percentage of pharmacists are in any one stage, what challenges or barriers have to be overcome to move from one stage to another, or what, if anything, is a significant emotional or intellectual event that would trigger a move, either quickly or slowly, into delivering enhanced levels of comprehensive pharmaceutical services.

The APhA–NWDA Concept Pharmacy is a practical and useful tool because it offers guidance in seven areas for those working through the first three stages of Prochaska's change model and find themselves ready to take action on:

- Workflow and facility redesign
- Communication
- Documentation
- Technology
- Marketing
- Education and training
- Money matters

These themes are echoed repeatedly in the pharmacists' stories told in Section II of this book, Uncommon People. In addition, Chapter 3 summarizes the key points from each of these seven areas and gives examples from the pharmacist profiles that follow. The goal of this book is simple. It provides insights that bridge the gap that exists when someone is contemplating practice change and is searching for some encouragement to take that first step.

The Concept Pharmacy resource is similar to a guide created in the early 1970s for the APhA's promotion of a new practice paradigm, then called the "office practice pharmacy." In this earlier project, the APhA developed a program for those who embraced a purely service-centered pharmacy that was free from commercialism. This meant a more professional-looking prescription center without a "front end" selling over-the-counter drugs and other commodities. Those who started such a practice and adhered to the APhA guidelines could earn a seal of approval from APhA attesting to their commitment. Office practice pharmacy may have been a concept far ahead of its time, but many who adopted this new style of practice found they had to retain some old-style community practices if they were to remain in business.

What was lacking then, as now, is practical advice on what kinds of new thinking and personal support systems it takes to assimilate and build a new professional paradigm, especially in community settings. We hope this book addresses this issue.

REFERENCES

1. Commission to Implement Change in Pharmaceutical Education: Maintaining Our Commitment to Change, American Association of Colleges of Pharmacy, Alexandria, VA, 1997.
2. Kennedy, D.T. et al., The role of academia in community based pharmaceutical care, *Pharmacotherapy*, 17(6), 1352–1356, 1997.
3. Johnson, J.A. and Bootman, J.L., Drug-related morbidity and mortality: a cost of illness model, *Arch. Intern. Med.*, 155, 1949–1956, 1995.
4. Johnson, J.L. and Bootman, J.L., Drug-related morbidity and mortality and the economic impact of pharmaceutical care, *Am. J. Health-Syst. Pharm.*, 54, 554–557, 1997.
5. Ernst, F.R. and Grizzle, A.J., Drug-related morbidity and mortality: updating the cost of illness model, *J. APhA*, 41, 192–199, 2001.
6. Fischer, L.R. et al., Pharmaceutical care and utilization in an HMO, *Eff. Clin. Pract.*, 5(2), 207–210, 2002.
7. Campbell, M. et al., Framework for design and evaluation of complex interventions to improve health, *Br. Med. J.*, 321, 694–696, 2000.
8. Rothman, R. and Weinberger, M., The role of pharmacists in clinical care: where do we go from here? *Eff. Clin. Pract.*, 5(2), 224–228 (www.acponline.org/journals/ecp/marapr02/rothman), 2002.
9. Currie, J.D. and Chrischilles, E.A., Effect of a training program on community pharmacists' detection of and intervention in drug-related problems, *J. Am. Pharm. Assoc.*, NS 37, 182–191, 1997.
10. Anon., *Principles of Practice for Pharmaceutical Care*, American Pharmaceutical Association, Washington, D.C., 1995.
11. Blunt, C.L., McKenny, J., and Czlarky, T., in *A Practical Guide to Pharmaceutical Care*, Rover, J.P., Haggerty, H.P., Currie, J.D. et al., Eds., American Pharmaceutical Association, Washington, D.C., 1998, chap. 3.
12. Hanne, H. et al., Improving drug therapy for patients with asthma, *J. Am. Pharm. Assoc.*, 41(4), 539–550, 2001.
13. Zellmer, W., Research to evaluate various methods and systems for the delivery of pharmaceutical care, *Am. J. Hosp. Pharm.*, 50, 1720–1723, 1993.
14. McDonough, R.D., Rovers, J.P., and Currie, J.D., Obstacles to the implementation of pharmaceutical care in the community setting, *J. Am. Pharm. Assoc.*, 38, 87–95, 1998.

15. The APhA/NWDA Concept Pharmacy Project, American Pharmaceutical Association and the National Wholesale Druggists Association, Washington, D.C., 1996 (now available from the Health Care Distributors and Manufacturers Association, Reston, VA).

16. Prochaska, J.D., DiClemente, C.C., and Norcross, J.C., In search of how people change, *Am. Psychol.*, 47, 1102–1114, 1997.

2

HEALTH CARE TRENDS DRIVING ENHANCED PHARMACY SERVICES

In spite of significant market uncertainty about pharmaceutical care as a business model, a number of trends and forces impacting health care support it. Innovative, enhanced, and value-added pharmaceutical care is also known as *medication therapy management services*.[1] After years of trying to achieve public understanding of effective pharmacy practice and as a new millennium begins with a nationwide shortage of pharmacists, organized pharmacy finally has the attention of a Congress that is looking to contain runaway prescription benefit costs. The APhA has proffered a simple, easily understood explanation of what pharmacists do best — improve patient outcomes and drug cost containment by providing medication therapy management services.

This definition of what pharmacists can, should, and will be doing is another attempt by the profession's leadership to state simply what direction the profession should be taking. This phrase is crafted under assumptions about what the market will support, assign value to, and, ultimately, for what it will compensate pharmacists. Fortunately, society has supported the value-added benefits of its pharmacists, but unfortunately it believes the services should be offered at no charge. Pharmacy has not been a complacent profession, however, and some of its risk-taking members have initiated and acted on new thinking about their business models.

New pharmacy business models are emerging as a result of a number of forces that impact not only pharmacy, but all health care professions. According to the HDMA's *Scanning Horizons 2001*[1] these forces include:

- The Internet
- Biotechnology
- Consumer activism (both in demand for services and their influence on public policy)
- Use of alternative and complementary therapies

In general, these forces are converging to exert continual pressure on today's business margins, driving firms to continually improve their operational efficiency or create more-differentiated, higher-valued product lines and services. This is the fundamental driving force behind competing and surviving in any U.S. health care business today. Pharmacy is responding to these pressures by making the dispensing process more efficient and by expanding patient-care services, such as those offered by the pharmacists presented in this book.

Three issues offer encouragement for pharmacy's survival and its business model. First, following a decade of decline, the National Community Pharmacists Association (NCPA) reports that the number of community pharmacies has grown for the second straight year, indicating demand and strength in new service offerings. Second, according to estimates from NCPA's National Institute for Pharmacist Care Outcomes (NIPCO), over 12,000 pharmacists have become credentialed through various pharmaceutical care programs. And third, the medication therapy management services model has been documented as a means to end medication errors. That said, the profession still faces enormous challenges because of its pharmacist shortage as well as time spent on issues involving third-party insurance coverage, including increased administrative duties. Thus, to offer new services, many pharmacists are looking to implement new technologies and systems that make the dispensing process less labor intensive and more convenient for patients. Their tactics include:

- Products packaged in unit-of-use to reduce labor costs
- Bar coding to reduce potential errors
- Central filling of prescriptions to reduce costs while improving care
- Central adjudication of third-party claims to reduce in-store administrative work
- Automated voice, computer, Internet, and other refill systems to improve workflow and customer service
- Electronic prescribing and routing to reduce errors and improve administration of refill approvals

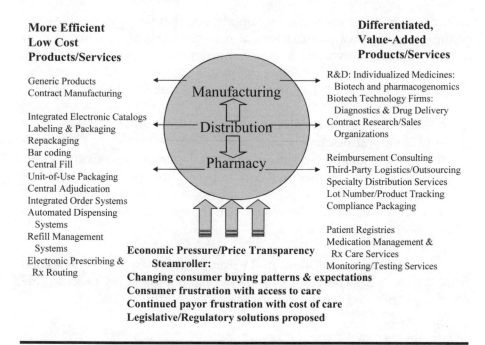

More Efficient Low Cost Products/Services

Differentiated, Value-Added Products/Services

Generic Products
Contract Manufacturing

Manufacturing

R&D: Individualized Medicines:
  Biotech and pharmacogenomics
Biotech Technology Firms:
  Diagnostics & Drug Delivery

Integrated Electronic Catalogs
Labeling & Packaging
Repackaging
Bar coding
Central Fill
Unit-of-Use Packaging
Central Adjudication
Integrated Order Systems
Automated Dispensing
  Systems
Refill Management
  Systems
Electronic Prescribing &
  Rx Routing

Distribution

Pharmacy

Contract Research/Sales
  Organizations

Reimbursement Consulting
Third-Party Logistics/Outsourcing
Specialty Distribution Services
Lot Number/Product Tracking
Compliance Packaging

Patient Registries
Medication Management &
  Rx Care Services
Monitoring/Testing Services

Economic Pressure/Price Transparency Steamroller:
Changing consumer buying patterns & expectations
Consumer frustration with access to care
Continued payor frustration with cost of care
Legislative/Regulatory solutions proposed

Figure 2.1 Industry response to major forces: transformation to new business models. (From Millonig, M., Castueble, T., and Heffner, S., *Scanning Horizons 2001*, Healthcare Distribution Management Association, Reston, VA, 2001. With permission.)

Challenges to these new technologies and process systems include the cost of implementing them and working with state regulators who are trying to keep pace with the impact on processes, procedures, personnel, and outcomes that they bring.

As they work to implement efficient operations systems, pharmacies are also creating a more profitable business model. According to *Scanning Horizons*,[1] what will continue to unfold is a model based on differentiation among pharmacy providers. Pharmacies will no longer look alike, but will evolve to meet the different needs of each community. They will also develop wellness models and bring alternative or complementary therapies into an integrated, holistic set of services. If not, pharmacists will risk having patients seek services and treatments elsewhere (Figure 2.1).

In support of a business model for medication management therapy services, or pharmaceutical care, is the influence brought by empowered consumers. Today's consumers are wiser, more knowledgeable, and, because of the Internet, are richly laden with information about diseases and their treatments. There is a fast-growing body of consumers who need help from someone willing to see that they get the best use of their medications, pharmaceutical care, or medication management therapy services, however each may be defined and delivered.

For pharmacists, then, a business model to conceptualize a patient-centered paradigm will require them to pay attention to:

- The market behavior of patients and the realities for what they will or will not pay[2]
- Their personal commitment to an easily articulated, easily understood, and accepted mission between the profession and the public
- Core competency necessary for the pharmacist to deliver on the promise of the new mission

Such a model can be illustrated using the analogy of a three-legged stool (Figure 2.2), where a new professional paradigm rests on a stable platform supported by three equal legs. These three legs are:

1. Market realities
2. Commitment to a simple, common mission
3. Competent pharmacists who work in harmony and support each other to earn public and professional trust, work collectively to improve value-added services, and find payment for improving patient-care outcomes

The stool analogy is used to illustrate that enhanced pharmacy service is more than an object upon which to sit. A stool provides a stable platform upon which one can stand and obtain a new perspective of pharmacy by being better able to see. Thus, any model used to illustrate pharmaceutical care should allow pharmacy to reinvent itself during turbulent times by bringing focus to its core competencies, mission, and market realities, and, to serve — as all economic and business models do — as a means of illustrating and testing a new model for doing something differently.

Models have the ability to illustrate the demand for medical services, such as pharmaceutical care, as they do for other goods and services in a market system. This is because pharmaceutical care helps to produce good health and creates social and economic utility. Because of its utility, pharmaceutical care has value. Anything with value-utility can be illustrated using a two-dimensional utility demand curve whose shape illustrates the relationship between the outcomes of a service or good and its inputs. Such a curve for pharmaceutical care illustrates

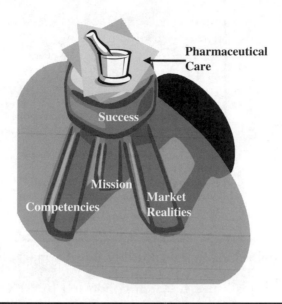

Pharmaceutical Care

Success

Mission

Market Realities

Competencies

Figure 2.2   A business model (paradigm) for enhanced pharmacist services.

that as outcomes increase, they occur at a decreasing rate of return. This means a pharmacist delivering comprehensive pharmaceutical services finds that due to the law of diminishing marginal productivity, each successive intervention creates a smaller improvement in health. Thus, each increase in health that a pharmacist is able to generate creates a smaller increase in the utility of pharmaceutical care[3] (Figure 2.3).

Consumers decide for which combination of goods and services, including pharmaceutical care, they are willing to pay. According to microeconomic theory, they will then choose a level of pharmaceutical care at which they perceive they are receiving the greatest value for their dollar, i.e., the level of maximum utility. The problem is that pharmaceutical care is difficult to measure and quantify because its service component has always been tied to the sale of a product. This is due to many reasons, including but not limited to:

■ Lack of uniformity in its early implementation
■ Variety of disease states for which services are offered
■ Limit in availability of comprehensive, nondisease-specific services
■ Lack of, or limited, documentation about where pharmaceutical care services are offered
■ Limited resources for funding studies

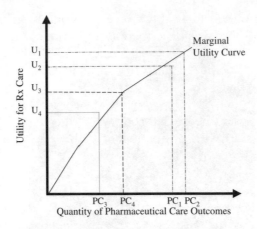

Figure 2.3 Diminishing marginal utility for pharmaceutical care.

Unpublished qualitative research conducted by APhA and NWDA during the course of their Concept Pharmacy Project confirmed that many consumers' and other health professionals' concerns eased once they were given a simpler and more focused description of pharmaceutical care services. That said, virtually all published surveys of consumers, and some anecdotal evidence from pharmacists, reveal that consumers will embrace and pay for pharmaceutical care services once they have an appreciation for what it is and how they can participate in it to achieve better health for themselves.

A 1996 APhA national pharmacy consumer survey conducted among 1200 household decision makers (68% female, 77% with some or all prescription costs paid by insurance, 75% with a prescription filled in the past 6 months, and 54% using chain pharmacies) found that:

■ Their traditional service expectations were being met, with more than 80% receiving written information and more than half receiving verbal information with their prescriptions.
■ They were highly loyal, with more than 50% using the same pharmacy for more than 5 years.
■ Although they want more information, 67% perceive pharmacists as too busy to provide it.
■ Of the total, 40% agreed it can be difficult to tell which person behind the prescription counter is the pharmacist.
■ It was important to some degree to 45% of respondents to have private consultation space available in the pharmacy.

Nearly 70% responded favorably or very favorably to the pharmaceutical care concept that was described as a pharmacist doing four things:

- Reviewing medical history and medications and developing a treatment plan
- Discussing the plan, answering questions about it and medications
- Recommending necessary changes in the plan
- Following up with the patient and the physician

What survey respondents liked about the concept was the double-checking of prescriptions and follow-up, having more information available, building a stronger relationship with the pharmacist, the interaction between the pharmacist and physician, and, finally, learning about medication side effects and interactions. Concerns were expressed about privacy of information and the cost, but fully 45% of those surveyed had no concerns at all.

What about their willingness to pay for services? Again, while many would like free services, more than one third would pay, preferring a monthly fee over an annual or per prescription fee. And, most importantly, despite being a loyal group, more than 31% would switch pharmacies in order to obtain these services. In spite of early innovative pharmacists who forged ahead to implement comprehensive pharmacy services without regard to payment, the fact is that there are many consumers willing to support and pay for pharmaceutical care. This is an important consideration for other pharmacists who are less risk-tolerant, but still want to provide an expanded service. For them the outlook is bright, but issues that must be addressed remain before pharmacists nationwide are paid for providing expanded services. These needs explain why the demand for pharmaceutical care today is still "fuzzy," and why the models and means to state that a competitive market price exists that will foster an equilibrium between demand and supply in a competitive system is an exercise in fuzzy math (Figure 2.4). These needs include:

- Researching and documenting positive outcomes associated with pharmaceutical care
- Seeking and gaining recognition as providers under Medicare
- Implementing collaborative practice in all states
- Creating the ability for pharmacists to immunize in all states
- Raising sufficient capital to implement new services

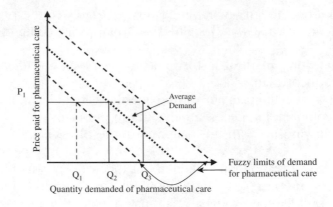

Figure 2.4 The fuzzy demand curve for pharmaceutical care.

■ Educating consumers and policy makers about the services and their benefits
■ Creating sufficient capacity to provide services when and where they are needed

Pharmaceutical care, medication management therapy services, and other professional paradigms should also be perceived as insurance policies for the profession of pharmacy. This is because they bring opportunities to manage risk in a turbulent market. This turbulence could obliterate a time-honored and respected profession if such market forces as managed care, third-party compensation, formulary management, aging populations, empowered consumers, three-, four-, and even five-tiered copays, Internet-based pharmacies, and risk-based contracts for defined populations were to dominate. All these issues are high-impact issues in health care. Additionally, the continued push for prescription payment based on actual acquisition cost and transparency in prescription pricing is contributing to downward margins in the "traditional" dispensing pharmacy business. Thus we suggest pharmaceutical care is a powerful construct to motivate and empower pharmacists to forge new and creative marketplace innovations and to stop a profession from becoming complacent.

Never be entirely idle, but either be reading, or writing, or praying, or meditating, or endeavoring something for the public good.

—Thomas à Kempis

The interviews in Part II are with pharmacists, who, although they may not recognize it, are helping to keep their profession from becoming complacent and perhaps disappear, as did suppliers of buggy whips when they failed to see the opportunities created by a better idea — the introduction of the automobile. We offer these interviews as inspiration for all pharmacists to deliver higher levels of patient care, and act on the advice of Peter Drucker who said, "When one reaches one's objective, it is not a time to celebrate but a time to do some new thinking."

REFERENCES

1. Millonig, M., Castueble, T., and Heffner, S., *Scanning Horizons 2001*, Healthcare Distribution Management Association, Reston, VA, 2001.
2. D'Angelo, A., We have never been stronger, *U.S. Pharm.*, 26(4), April, 2, 2001, p. 2.
3. Samuelson, P.A., *Introduction to Economics*, 17th ed., McGraw-Hill College Division, New York, 2001, p. 19.

3

BUILDING INNOVATION INTO YOUR PRACTICE: SEVEN COMPONENTS OF CHANGE

How does one begin a pharmaceutical care practice? While you may wish to communicate better with physicians and patients, you must be motivated and active in managing medications and educating people about improving their health. Although getting paid for doing what provides professional satisfaction — giving better care — is certainly a benefit, change under any circumstances is difficult, even painful. Not only do you have to change how you see yourself, you have to change how others see you too.

Adding pharmaceutical care services may sound time-consuming and labor intensive, but it is not. In this chapter we outline the steps you can follow to bring the kind of changes to pharmacy practice that make you an active, trusted partner in the management of patient care. While implementing these steps, you will also:

- Keep learning and growing in your work
- Create more satisfying relationships with people in your workplace and community
- Make more money

In researching innovative pharmacy care, we found certain techniques and new ideas showing up again and again and thus developed the following set of seven guiding principles. These principles came out of work we did originally for the Concept Pharmacy project,[1] the

Herculean collaborative effort of the NWDA and the APhA.* The project helped pharmacists and others understand the benefits of patient-focused care and highlighted the best practices of innovators in pharmacy from around the country. As part of this work we conducted a survey of practicing pharmacists who were incorporating pharmaceutical care into their professional lives, and from that work distilled their insights into seven guiding elements:

- Workflow and facility design
- Communication with physicians and patients
- Documentation of practice interventions
- Application of new technology
- Marketing strategies
- Education and training
- Financial affairs

Not everyone we talked to addressed every one of these seven guiding principles to the same extent. We found these principles to be the collective keys that opened the doors to their ability to implement an active model of pharmaceutical care.

WORKFLOW AND FACILITY DESIGN

The goal of patient-centered pharmaceutical care is to improve the quality of patients' lives by identifying and resolving drug therapy problems. To accomplish this, pharmacists must have their priorities set and utilize their time efficiently, so that tasks not directly related to patient care will not interfere with visualizing the patient's entire health picture and the focus will not be solely on the medications being dispensed.

In our work we heard stories akin to the following as being a typical event in a community pharmacy. It is 5:45 p.m., and a long line of people, tired after a day's work, has formed in front of the prescription counter at the back of a drugstore. People fidget, small children knock into adults, as the pharmacist and her assistant try to fill a growing number of prescriptions. The person at the front of the

---

* The summary that forms this chapter was based on the APhA/NWDA Concept Pharmacy Project's Workbook, *Planning Your Journey to Patient-Focused Care*. It is being used here with the permission of the American Pharmaceutical Association, the National Wholesale Druggists Association, and the Healthcare Distributors and Manufacturers Association.

line is getting frustrated, perhaps challenging the price or finding that his insurer has refused to pay for his prescription. "But I'm going out of town tonight for three weeks and I need this prescription!" "Your insurance company won't pay for this refill until Monday, I'm sorry." "Well, how much will it cost if I just pay for it myself?" "Probably over a hundred dollars if you pay without insurance." "Ridiculous! Tell them...." Meanwhile, more people join the line and shoppers looking for cough syrup or greeting cards try to edge past the crowd in back or elbow their way through the line. Already tired, people begin to get irritable and roll their eyes, shaking their heads at each other. Everyone's nerves begin to fray, including those of the assistant and the pharmacist. Such a scenario is a no-win situation for all because no one has taken a holistic look at workflow, customer traffic patterns, space constraints, task functions, and how customer-patients are treated. By taking a look at the entire pharmacy and the staff functions within it, pharmaceutical-care professionals have found creative ways to add services within limited space and time constraints.

In a traditional community pharmacy, a patient usually presents a prescription to a clerk or technician. The pharmacist checks for warning notices, obtains refill authorizations when necessary, fills the prescription, and performs a final check before returning the medication to a clerk or technician, who gives it to the patient and accepts payment. In most cases any information given is drug specific, and to meet the requirements of the Omnibus Budget Reconciliation Act of 1990 (OBRA 1990), the drug information is stapled to the prescription bag as a leaflet. Successful patient-focused practice will shift staff patterns. For example, a clerk or technician will greet the patient and capture important initial demographic information. The technician retrieves the patient's chart, gives it to the pharmacist, and enters the prescription information into the computer. The technician also alerts the pharmacist to any warning notices. The technician fills the prescription and gives it to the pharmacist for the final check. During this process, the pharmacist meets with the patient to discuss his or her understanding of the medication and to check for any drug therapy problems. The pharmacist frequently has an arrangement with the prescriber and, on behalf of the patient, ensures optimal and effective medication selection and management.

Redesigning pharmacy workflow and facilities sends a clear message to your customers (i.e., patients, administrators, other health care professionals, payers) that you are committed to a new way of practicing pharmacy. As you consider redesigning your pharmacy, talk with

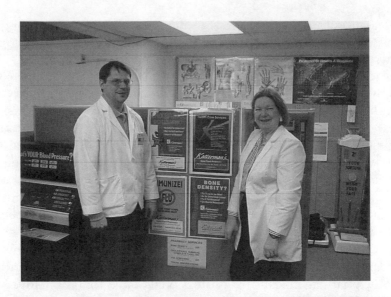

In the separate professional services area, John and Beverly Schaefer show off Bev's innovative pharmacy design.

colleagues and pharmacy innovators to find out what has worked for them. Involve your staff and ask for their input. One example of a successful reassessment of store space and staffing may be found in Beverly Schaefer's concept.

Schaefer hired a designer to create a new floor plan for the store. By splitting the front-end merchandise away from the prescription area and reorienting the aisles of the store from a straight front-to-back design to an innovative diagonal design, she created a pleasant ambience for her customers and one where they will know if they are in the general merchandise area or in the professional services area. Thus attractively displayed, upscale merchandise focuses general traffic at one end of the store, and her well-staffed pharmacy, operating under extended hours, allows for a good flow of patients through that area. This well-thought-out floor plan ensures an efficient use of space, while her choice of additional staff members — often students rather than technicians — has proved to be pleasing to her clientele.

Believing in the importance of empowering the consumer, Max Peoples emphasizes counseling in his practice. His strategy for redesign was to make room in his pharmacy for two private counseling areas paneled in mahogany, separated from the dispensing area. By doing so, he created a place where patients can speak with ease with a pharmacist about their care. Their privacy is protected, and they feel they are receiving close personal attention; further, these arrangements keep the flow undisturbed in the high traffic area by the dispensing and purchase areas.

Greg Wedin's pharmacy was among a group of 20 pharmacies in Minnesota selected to participate in the seminal Minnesota Pharmaceutical Care Project. Pharmacist and pharmaceutical care theory co-creator, Linda Strand, Ph.D., directed this project through the University of Minnesota's College of Pharmacy Peters Institute. Its purpose was to create the care process often associated with pharmaceutical care. Strand and fellow author Dr. Charles Hepler wrote a 1990 paper on a pharmacist's ability to solve drug therapy problems. Their paper documented comprehensive pharmacy services provided to a group of Blue Cross/Blue Shield (BC/BS) patients. The study identified whether any of the eight categories of drug-related problems, outlined by Strand and Hepler, existed and what interventions resolve them. Bitten by a desire to "do more" than getting involved in the project, Greg Wedin made changes to his pharmacy's layout and workflow. He separated the prescription entry and pickup areas, having pharmacists staff the prescription pickup in order to conduct the initial interview with patients and get any needed information to help further in any drug therapy management decisions. Technicians did the actual filling of prescriptions, with the pharmacists providing the final check, managing the drug utilization review (DUR) process, and giving prescriptions back to patients. This arrangement expedited his workflow, and gave the pharmacists an opportunity for a one-on-one encounter with the patients, along with all the benefits of improved communication that accrue to both.

COMMUNICATING WITH PHYSICIANS AND PATIENTS

Providing patient-focused care places additional demands on the need for effective and efficient communication skills on pharmacists and staff. In addition, the quality of the relationship and communication between patient and pharmacist has been shown to be a key ingredient in patient compliance with drug therapy plans. Good communication skills, such as showing empathy, listening to what patients say, and paying attention to their concerns, demonstrate caring to patients. These skills enhance the patient–pharmacist relationship. They also help patients to see their pharmacists as competent, trustworthy, and caring.

Here is a story that might have ended differently had the pharmacist shown better communication skills. A listless young woman comes into a pharmacy to have her thyroid replacement medication prescription refilled. She hesitantly tries to strike up a conversation with the pharmacist, who is taking care of some important paperwork. He truly is interested in listening to her, but he feels pressured to complete his work, so he is trying to multitask. The young woman is concerned about her thyroid replacement therapy. She begins to murmur something about feeling very washed out. She wants to explain to the pharmacist that she had started some supplements, but they don't seem to help. But he is not looking at her and he is half-turned toward his desk. She thinks, "Oh, he must think I am just complaining." So, she stops talking and goes away. Neither of them realizes that her herbal supplements are interfering with absorption of her thyroid medicine — she, because she does not know about this effect and he, because he does not know the patient is mixing drugs. Had the patient not became discouraged before she told him her story, she would have communicated this important piece of information.

Communication with all customer-patients is important. Depending on the situation, your message may be one of counseling patients about the use of medications, educating payers about the benefits of patient-focused care, or informing physicians about drug therapy problems experienced by their patients. Providing patient-focused care also requires that you collect more information in greater depth from patients and share more information with others. In each case, you must consider the most appropriate delivery method. Will it be a face-to-face conversation, telephone call, personal letter, reminder service, or some combination?

Pharmacist Rick Mohall's communication skills were an asset when his company joined forces with BC/BS of Western Pennsylvania in 1999 in a test of the impact of pharmaceutical care services on their Medicare patients. Rick was approached to participate in developing the pilot program because of his reputation as a "doer" with regard to patient care. Always seeking ways to talk with seniors and others in his community about medication management, health care promotion, and other pharmacy topics, Mohall was also an active participant in neighborhood health fairs and screenings.

Speaking about his work making the changes necessary to offer more active patient care, he remarks:

> I've always enjoyed interacting with people and have found it fun to take the initiative to be involved in ways that I can communicate with patients.... We found whatever space we could to provide counseling, whether it was moving chairs into the pharmacy aisles or finding space

in the back room somewhere. It didn't matter. We did whatever we had to do to make it work. I truly believe the key is for a patient to have a one-on-one relationship with the pharmacist.

The written word is also an effective way to establish and maintain lines of communication. Some of your patients may be more comfortable with written consultations than with direct contact; thus it is good to always follow up on meetings with patients by sending them letters summarizing your consultation. It is especially helpful with elderly people who may have difficulties remembering detailed material and appreciate the support of a written follow-up.

Elderly patients are appreciative of telephone calls; they are often isolated and must juggle many medications. It may be difficult for them to get transportation and thus they may see their doctors infrequently. Pharmacists are being looked upon as their advocates and helpmates who provide a needed service by helping them better manage their medication. They also are delighted to know you care, and can become strongly loyal patients, spreading the word to their friends and family. Many other people who are homebound or otherwise isolated by medical conditions appreciate and benefit from a caring touch by telephone — new mothers, women with sick children, those recovering from surgery. The telephone can be a lifeline, both figuratively and literally, for such people. As their pharmacist, you can do a lot of good by staying in touch and showing you care.

Restructuring your practice to provide a more active model of patient care depends on engaging your staff in taking on more responsibilities. In order to do this you will need to build good communication with co-workers as well. As Kim Swiger states, "Explain what you're doing and why to colleagues at your practice and other sites. To succeed, pharmaceutical care requires teamwork."

Judy Hanson's experience in her practice illustrates this point. In 1996, Dominick's, the pharmacy where she works, and Dr. Richard Hutchison of the University of Chicago College of Pharmacy began to explore ways of implementing pharmaceutical care programs. Dominick's offers programs for patients on a range of subjects, including asthma, diabetes, hypertension, hyperlipidemia, smoking cessation, osteoporosis, immunizations, and nutrition-wellness. Hanson's strength in building interpersonal relationships has been key to her ability to implement these programs. "Educating the pharmacy staff on the vision — what we were trying to do and how it would change their work — was the first thing we did. They were very receptive, although a lot of reassurance was required." Initially nervous assistants can get a shot of empowerment by seeing their job descriptions include more responsible work. Hanson got an enthusiastic buy-in from several members of her staff by enrolling them at no charge in programs having to do with their own health conditions.

Working collaboratively with physicians is essential to the long-term success of your pharmaceutical care practice. Richmond area pharmacist Michelle Shibley calls it a key component for the long-term success of her programs. She suggests that you "stay in touch with physicians by faxing a follow-up note from the pharmacist on each patient as [you] see them." Other approaches include sending summary letters to physicians regarding patients about whose medications you may have questions or comments and short visits or telephone calls to introduce your services to specialists in the area. When they see that you want to support their work, not challenge their authority, they will come to appreciate and depend on your services.

Certain specific techniques are recognized as good communication builders. Whether you are talking with staff members, physicians, patients, or payers, you open up better lines of communication with people by

■ Asking open-ended questions
■ Listening actively
■ Offering reflective responses

Finally, in your interactions with patients, physicians, and payers, being active in finding new opportunities to expand your pharmaceutical care services works well. Opportunities arise from one of three circumstances:

■ A new patient comes to you to get a prescription filled
■ A returning patient comes to get a refill of a maintenance medication
■ Anyone can come in and ask you a question about health, self-care, or a medication

Example: Pharmacist confirming a prescription with a physician

Situation: One of your pharmacists calls a physician to confirm the details of a prescription. During the conversation, the physician states that she hasn't been able to get the patient's blood pressure under control.

Opportunity: Tell the physician about your blood pressure monitoring service. Then follow up with a phone call, a personal letter, and possibly a face-to-face with a brochure describing the service and its benefits for patients and physicians.

The more clearly you envision your new, active role in patient health care, the more frequently you will see openings for the skills you offer. Be creative, be open to others and their needs. Always be ready to serve others as a professional and you will be surprised at the opportunities you will find for your services.

DOCUMENTING YOUR SERVICES

A young, enthusiastic pharmacist decides to offer individual consultations to patients with multiple medications. He posts a notice at a community center nearby. Several days later, a group of elderly patients come in together — they've just come from a bingo game and are going back to their apartment complex together. Taken off guard, not quite ready, he rushes around, gets some chairs, and interviews them, writing down what they tell him on a loose sheet of paper. He closes each consultation by promising to send them reminder letters. They are pleased and say they will tell their friends. After they leave, he feels pleased and happy. Their smiles warmed his heart. The young pharmacist feels great until he looks at his notes; he can't separate out the individual cases. There had been a pair of twins named Eleanor and Abbie (one takes cholesterol medicine, and the other takes Paxil). He doesn't remember which was which. There were two men named John (one has diabetes, the other Parkinson's), and three other men introduced themselves all at once. He thinks they are Morris, Tom, and Mort. From his scrawl, he isn't sure which is Morris' write-up and which is Mort's. He is aghast. How will he write up their letters? He squirms, realizing he will have to call them and ask them all over again.

Pharmacists are care-giving professionals. If expanded services are to be a mainstream part of your professional life, you must document and keep records that such services were in fact rendered.

In most pharmacies documentation systems verify the dispensing of a product where the pharmacist gathers information, such as for whom the prescription has been written, contact information, the use of other prescription medications, and allergies that might cause problems. Often a pharmacist is not certain why a given medication is prescribed. To provide enhanced patient care, a more holistic view is necessary and thus more information about the patient and his or her health condition is needed.

Patient-focused care requires more than simple documentation of patient data. The data require information management systems and processes in order to:

■ Collect and manage patient data
■ Monitor patient progress and health outcomes
■ Record and track billing and collection
■ Share information with the physician

This requires three interconnected databases:

1. For patient information
2. For follow-up, scheduling appointments, and reminders
3. For auditing billing and payment

Choices must be made between what is on paper and what is housed in computer-based systems. While data systems may sound intimidating or complex, they don't have to be. Start with what you already have on hand. Items as simple as a filing cabinet and forms that can be written on and photocopied are a good start. While you may eventually come to use sophisticated computer software and other technology, it all starts with a pencil, a piece of paper, and some common sense questions.

A first step is to assess how you handle patient information in your current practice. Take a look at your current documentation process. Do you use a paper- or computer-based system? Are you satisfied with it? Who enters the information and maintains it, you or an assistant? Does this approach seem efficient and reliable? How do you ensure the confidentiality of your patient information? Finally, do you think your current system can support the kinds of information needs you will place on it by practicing patient care? What changes might you consider making?

Providing patient-focused care shifts the requirements for documentation and information management as the priorities of the practice itself shift. If improving overall health of your patients becomes your new focus, the spotlight then is on identifying health care problems and solving them with appropriate drug therapy interventions. Pharmacy records are moving toward the medical model in that they become more problem-oriented under the pharmaceutical care approach. This means that the next step is to bolster prescription filing with patient care plans. A pharmaceutical care plan evolves from your assessment of the problem and describes the strategy or strategies to resolve it. You will find that as you develop care plans, you will produce communications for other audiences, e.g., physicians, third-party payers. Typically, a patient-focused pharmacy record includes the following information:

- Patient's medical problems and medications taken, including all prescriptions, OTC, and CAM (complementary and alternative medications)
- Drug therapy problems (adverse affects, overdose, underutilization)
- Steps taken to resolve the problems
- Prescriber and insurance information
- Emergency contact information

These areas comprise the basics of the information you need to make your patient's care plan complete. You should also record why the patient came to see you and how he or she described the problem. Include your analysis of the problems, outcomes of your interaction with the patient, and your follow-up plans. It may seem like a lot of extra work at first, but collecting and using this material about your patients will show them to you in a new light, within the context of their overall health condition. By the same token, working with your patients in this way will help them see you in a new light as well, i.e., as a professional concerned with them as people, someone who knows them, is paying attention to them, and cares about their well-being.

There are, of course, many ways of documenting information and interventions. You may want to come up with your own format or look to a professionally developed one. One of the common ways to keep information is in the Subjective, Objective Assessment Plan (SOAP) format.[2] Essentially, this is a form blocking out areas for input of basic information (name, date, type of visit), subjective comments, objective information, your assessment, care plan, and notes about follow-up. Pharmacist Diane Schultz sets an example for using this format. She is instituting a diabetes program at several stores in her pharmacy group. The plan is to structure the program with an appointment system, offering appointments several days a week during pharmacist shift overlap in the middle of the afternoon. Schultz plans to use SOAP (Figure 3.1) to document the interviews, and eventually bill for them using HCFA 1500 forms.

As you prepare to handle an increased volume of information you will need to address how to gather, store, and manage this information. As you think about capturing information, ask yourself:

- What vehicle will you use to gather information? You can use a pharmacist interview form, a checklist of key questions to ask each patient, or a patient questionnaire.
- How will you capture the information? Will the pharmacist or an assistant perform the interviews? Who will review the form with patients and check for completeness?

In thinking about storing patient information, ask yourself:

- How will patient data be stored?
- Will it be a paper- or computer-based system?
- What software application will you use?
- How will you back up your data?
- How will you ensure confidentiality in the maintenance of the records?

Finally, you must think in terms of the entire flow of the information through your system, no matter how modest. Take a couple of steps back in your mind and look at the whole picture at your facility. Ask yourself:

- Who will be responsible for inputting and retrieving patient data? How will you be able to retrieve the information efficiently?
- What kind of system will you put in place to monitor patients' follow-up needs? Will it be you or another person?
- Who will manage the billing and collection procedures? Will you have to hire someone? What person already on staff has some medical office experience? Can you afford to hire a student or intern to help with this work? Where will you find them?

Do not put a lot of pressure on yourself to create an elaborate system until you are ready and need it. Start simple, start slow, start with pen and paper. As you develop your forms and processes, keep checking to make sure that they are easy to use for both staff and patients and that they ask for information clearly. Test them with

Diabetes Visit Summary (SOAP)

Patient Name: _____ Date: _____

Patient's Primary Complaint: (S) _____

_____

_____

Objective Findings: (O) _____

_____

_____

Assessment: (A) _____

_____

_____

_____

Consulted Patient On:

___ Diabetes Overview	___ Medication	___ Foot Care
___ Blood Glucose Monitoring	___ Insulin	___ Cholesterol/BP
___ Interpreting SBGM Results	___ Hypoglycemia	___ Sick Days
___ Nutrition	___ Hyperglycemia	___ Community Resources
___ Exercise	___ Chronic Complications	___ Other: _____

Plan: (P)

___ SMBG Recommendations: _____

_____

_____

___ Insulin/Medication Recommendations: _____

_____

_____

___ Exercise Recommendations: _____

_____

___ Complications/Self-Care Recommendations _____

_____

_____

___ Other Recommendations/Notes: _____

_____

_____

Follow-Up Scheduled For: _____ Referred To: _____

_____ Time Spent with Patient: _____ minutes
Pharmacist's Signature

Figure 3.1 Diane Schultz's modified SOAP formats.

friends and family, or colleagues. Ask for feedback from your patients. And be very careful with the information you gather; they are legal documents. Have every entry signed and dated; guard the integrity and confidentiality of these documents. Never delete, only add information.

This increased care taken with documentation will pay off in tangible terms. In the case of managed care, third-party payers or clients require proof of medical necessity and proof of service delivery. Good documentation will meet those needs. This augmented documentation and improved information management will position you as a health care provider, not just a dispenser of medications.

There is no right or wrong way. You have to just try an approach, and if it doesn't work, try another. Judy Hanson again serves as a great example. When her pharmacies began to document new pharmaceutical care services, they initially used a commercially available software system but, says Hanson, "[we] found it too laborious, especially since it wasn't integrated with the dispensing system. Now, we document by hand, and I believe that really helps the pharmacist understand the pharmaceutical care process. We use templates with standard formats and flowcharts to put things in SOAP note format." They use a fee structure for services based on the resource-based relative value scale (RBRVS).

On the other hand, Tina Lampe-Izaguirre and her colleague Karen Halvorsen have opted for a commercial software solution. They were recruited several years ago to plan and implement the Eckerd Patient Care Center. One of their decisions was to document care using a patient-centered pharmaceutical care software from a commercial vendor.

You may even find it useful to devise your own materials. Beverly Schaefer created her own solution for documentation in the form of a very creative at-a-glance text/graphic tool. It compiles useful, meaningful information, and is easy to interpret. Her pharmacy sends the results to patient physicians with a cover letter. An additional payoff to this skillful documentation is that it brings the physicians on board. Beverly notes, "We learned early on, if you take a public health approach to the services you are providing, physicians have a hard time arguing against them."

USING NEW TECHNOLOGY

The following is a scenario that is not as unlikely as it may seem. Two pharmacists, partners in practice, decide to offer a series of programs for patients with diabetes, high blood pressure, and asthma. They write up some ideas and information, and hire a local print shop to design and publish 1000 brochures. They get the brochures printed on glossy paper. They seem fine at first, but upon closer inspection are disappointing. The names are misspelled, the wrong location is given, and the bill comes to $2000. The pharmacists are aghast. Their assistant is standing nearby and hears the conversation. She has been helping her daughter's Girl Scout troop sell cookies for the last 2 years and has been designing the flyers for them on her home PC. "I wish you had told me," she said. "I could have done it for you for free. I have software at home that can help design flyers. You would only have to pay for the printing, probably just a couple of hundred dollars." They look at each other and groan. Using new user-friendly technology, the pharmacists could have accomplished their objectives more cost-effectively.

As you increase patient-focused activities, you may find that your current office equipment and communication materials are insufficient. Examine your office tools and determine whether they are going to remain sufficient for your needs. Technology can help you run your pharmacy practice more efficiently and let you spend more time focusing on patient care than on paperwork. It can also help you communicate and network with others, learn about the latest research results, and organize and plan your time more efficiently.

It can be challenging trying to determine which technological advances are right for your practice. You might feel tempted to buy the latest gadget being promoted, but a good way to resist this temptation is to focus on the goals of your practice. Make technology your slave — don't be a slave to it. Start by listing the goals you want to achieve and then find the technology to achieve them. Try to find one device that will be useful in several areas. Don't overlook low-tech tools either. Tools such as checklists, worksheets, decision tables, and algorithms enhance staff performance. Paper-based planning and organizing systems, such as personal organizers, planners, and filing systems can also be very effective and cost-efficient. Be sure that you and your staff receive adequate training on each new piece of technology. No system works well run by undertrained users. Look to your current staff and assess their expertise. You may have someone on staff who is proficient in a given area and can teach others.

Technology can help manage several areas of your practice. These areas can be grouped around the telephone, computer hardware and software, time-management systems, and other technical tools.

Depending on your particular situation, some or all of these will be very helpful:

- Fax machine to send and receive prescriptions and other communications
- Pager to maintain your accessibility
- Answering machine
- Multiple phone lines
- Cell phone
- Computer software for word processing, to create databases, run money management and desktop publishing programs
- Time management systems to help you perform planning and scheduling functions
- Modem connection for Internet, e-mail, and professional and scientific information on the Web

You may also find it useful to have a laptop computer equipped with a modem for access to data and e-mail to take with you when traveling. Other useful technical equipment and tools that can help you with patient care are:

- Dictation equipment
- TV and VCR for educational videos
- Monitoring equipment for particular conditions (e.g., glucose testing equipment for diabetes)
- Educational materials and compliance aids
- Automatic pill counters and robotics
- Changeable lighted signs
- Individual beepers

In our interviews with successful pharmaceutical care practitioners, we saw a wide range of inventive uses of technological aids. Max Peoples has created a bar code scanning device used to match a prescription product's NDC code to the bottle of medication as it is actually dispensed. Peoples notes:

Every pharmacist dreads the day he or she dispenses the wrong medication. Some research shows 2% of all prescriptions are subject to errors. I can show it is as much as 7% in my store and that I have the tool to reduce or eliminate 75% of the mismatches between NDC numbers on the dispensing bottle and the prescription's product. It is very satisfying to me to know that I can help pharmacists ascertain they have the ointment in their hand when it should be the cream. These are errors to us, but are usually not realized as possibilities by the patient.

At Richmond Apothecaries, Michelle Shibley and her colleagues also have developed their own approach to customizing workplace tools for pharmaceutical care practice. Tightly integrating service with the dispensing process, they focus on this process to build a patient-care base and to identify program participants during their visits. They have devised a method to code patient records in the dispensing system so the pharmacist filling the prescription can identify the patient as part of a care program, creating concise, meaningful, and disease-specific evaluation tools for the pharmacist to use during these visits. They have further tailored available technology to their own needs. They have not found their pharmaceutical care software program as useful as a Microsoft Access database applied to meet their specialized in-house needs for documentation purposes.

Only you can determine which technological aids best suit your practice. Some will be invaluable; others you would never miss. And, like the pharmacists we met, you may develop your own.

DEVELOPING MARKETING STRATEGIES

Deciding to offer pharmaceutical care is only the first step in developing a service program. Patients will need to fully experience pharmaceutical care in order to understand why you are doing it and why they will benefit. In order for patients to experience these services, you need to get the message out to current patients, new patients, administrators, clients, other health care professionals, and the community at large. There is no best strategy for marketing pharmaceutical care. The message and the method depend on the services you are providing, your customers, your market, and what is best for your own particular practice.

For someone with no marketing background this task may seem daunting. Our advice is to start small and build on your experience and success. First, take time to analyze your practice and market. As you develop marketing materials, create a solid foundation, perhaps with a brochure describing services and fees. Distribute the brochure in the store and mail it to current customers. Over time, add additional strategies, such as personal visits with physicians, mass mailings, and presentations at the local library and community center. Talk with colleagues to find out what has worked for them. Evaluate what others have used to help you develop and refine your message. Easy-to-use software packages can help create your own marketing materials. Also explore other resources for marketing assistance, such as your wholesaler.

You can find many opportunities to market pharmaceutical care services in your practice. For example:

- Creating descriptive brochures
- Conducting in-store health screenings
- Sending personal letters
- Visiting physicians
- Sending out mass mailings
- Participating in health fairs
- Publishing a newsletter
- Giving lectures and presentations to various civic groups
- Offering wellness classes

Pharmacist Eric Graf has made excellent use of newsletters and seminars as marketing and educational tools at Ritzman's Pharmacy. A bimonthly newsletter is mailed to all patients and providers. The newsletters market Ritzman's natural product education seminars at four of their eight locations. Each seminar is open to the entire community and lasts about an hour. These seminars include natural hormone replacement therapy, cooking with soy, Yoga, cholesterol management, diabetes management, and stress management. In addition the pharmacy's brochure clearly states its goals (Figure 3.2).

Diane Schultz uses a different strategy to market a new outpatient immunization program. Her team's plans are to advertise the new service through newspaper ads, health education flyers to the community, direct mail, and by visiting people. They do physician education and awareness building through lunch meetings and direct mail.

Our mission is to provide comfort, security, and care in filling the needs of our customers with quality products, professional excellence, and service beyond the commonplace

---

Figure 3.2 The mission of Ritzman's Pharmacy.

As you see, marketing strategies vary, depending on the nature of the practice and the location, as well as the particular services offered. Tina Lampe-Izaguirre and her colleague Karen Halvorsen had a mandate to organize the Eckerd Patient Care Centers. They began with a series of brochures describing both the comprehensive services they planned to offer, as well as some with a disease-specific orientation. Building a patient base required time. Lampe-Izaguirre and Halvorsen concentrated on personally visiting physicians as well as pharmacists at surrounding Florida Eckerd stores to explain their services. They also were able to target their efforts by working with the corporate office to identify patients who might be good candidates for the new services. "We worked hard to build relationships with the store managers and pharmacists and presented our services at the Center as part of a team approach to helping patients. In addition to visiting every pharmacist at every store, we provided training to pharmacists at district meetings and our efforts were well received. As a result, referrals began coming to the Center from the stores."

Some things work; others don't. One pharmacy offered a hypertension control service as being a relatively simple way to start. It developed a pamphlet to market the service to patients and physicians, faxed the brochure to the physicians, and followed up by phone. A $20 per month fee was charged for four weekly appointments and unlimited blood pressure readings. While there was a lot of interest, many people did not think the service justified the expense and it was difficult getting it off the ground. The service was then changed to having a free blood pressure monitoring machine in each store instead. Being adaptable and learning the needs of your particular market will ensure that you gain successful acceptance of your services.

For Kim Swiger, marketing services to internal staff, patients, and physicians has been essential. She notes that explaining the new services to staff was an important start. "We needed to help store managers, employees, and pharmacy technicians understand how the services could help patients and the company." Her group instituted a variety of ways to reach people that may be candidates for pharmaceutical care services. A monthly customer newsletter, *Great News*, featured a piece focusing on nutrition and health. Blood pressure, cholesterol, lipid, glucose, hemoglobin, and bone density screenings at area stores were advertised in local newspapers (Figure 3.3). In addition to direct marketing through newsletters and letters to patients, they posted 2-week screening schedules at the stores.

MONDAY	TUESDAY	WEDNESDAY	THURSDAY	FRIDAY	SATURDAY
8 WELLNESS DAY Petersberg 10am-2pm	**9** WELLNESS DAY Fredericksberg 2pm-5pm Chippenham Crossing 2pm-4pm Colonial Heights 1pm-4pm Stony Point 1pm-4pm Laburnum 1pm-4pm ***Williamsburg 9:30am-1pm	**10** WELLNESS DAY Joe's Market 10am-4pm Mechanicsville 11am-3pm Ashland 11am-3pm	**11** WELLNESS DAY Brook Run 10am-2pm Patterson 1pm-3pm Short Pump 10am-2pm Chesterfield Towne Center 9am-2pm	**12** WELLNESS DAY Virginia Center Marketplace 9am-2pm *Chesterfield Meadows 9am-4pm *Westpark 9am-4pm	**13** *Blood Pressure Screenings by Convalescent Care **Screenings Sponsored by HCA Hospitals ***Sponsored by Williamsberg Community Hospital
15 **Screening Charges** Blood Pressure - FREE Cholesterol/HDL - $15 Full Lipid Profile - $25 Blood Glucose - $7 Hemoglobin A1c - $20 Bone Density - $25. **Available during scheduled Wellness Days** at Brook Run, Mechanicsville, Habour Pointe, Patterson and Short Pump.	**16** WELLNESS DAY Williamsberg 2pm-4pm Fredericksberg 2pm-5pm Colonial Heights 10am-2pm Stony Point 1pm-4pm Laburnum 1pm-4pm **BLOOD PRESSURE ONLY** *StaplesMill/Dumbarton 10am-1pm *Bermuda Square 10am-1pm	**17** WELLNESS DAY Joe's Market 10am-4pm Mechanicsville 11am-3pm Ashland 11am-3pm	**18** WELLNESS DAY Brook Run 10am-2pm FountainSquare 1pm-4pm Short Pump 10am-2pm Chesterfield Towne Center 9am-2pm **BLOOD PRESSURE ONLY** Chesterfield Meadows 10am-2pm **TRIGGER POINT MASSAGE** Virginia Center Marketplace 4pm-6pm	**19** WELLNESS DAY Virginia Center Marketplace 9am-2pm **Patterson 12pm-7pm **Carytown 12pm-7pm	**20** WELLNESS DAY **StaplesMill/Dumbarton 10am-3pm Oxbridge Square 10am-3pm **WOMEN'S HEALTH CHECK & OSTEOPOROSIS SCREENINGS** Short Pump 10am-3pm

Figure 3.3 Kim Swiger's newspaper ad for screenings.

You can save yourself time and increase your chances of success by developing a well-focused marketing plan following these steps:

- Analyze your market
- Identify competitors
- Determine your services
- Differentiate yourself from the competition
- Identify potential marketing strategies
- Select marketing strategies
- Create marketing materials
- Evaluate and revise the marketing plan

Each of these steps entails a process of analysis and change to tailor them to your own practice. Many resources are available to help you with this aspect of your practice. A well-conceived and executed plan can be the key to successful implementation of your new pharmaceutical care services. Take the time to study what you can comfortably offer, what people in your area need, and how you can make yourself stand out. Review all the steps if necessary.

INCORPORATING EDUCATION AND TRAINING INTO YOUR PRACTICE

To successfully incorporate patient-focused care into your practice, you need to ensure that you and your staff learn new skills. Everyone will need new perspectives and attitudes. Depending on the audience, this education may involve on-the-job training, seminars and certificate courses, self-study material, videos, informational brochures, pamphlets, and other marketing materials. The integration of patient-focused care requires that you turn your pharmacy into a learning organization. You and your partners should be continually reviewing workflow, systems, products and services, and customers. Assessing new educational and training needs and determining how to meet them will be an ongoing process. Continual advances in drug therapy and technology will require that you continue to acquire new skills and information to continue to give the best care to your patients.

Once you've made the decision to implement patient-focused care, begin your education and training efforts immediately. Studies have shown that it takes 3 to 4 months for technicians to become proficient in dispensing and for everyone to become comfortable in their new roles.[3] As you train your technicians in dispensing, verify the transfer of learning to the job. Closely observe their work for a period of time until you have confidence in their grasp of their new skills.

Involve your staff as much as possible throughout the implementation process. Ask them for their input and assistance. They will add valuable perspectives and their involvement will create buy-in for the changes. New job descriptions can help everyone focus on their new roles and responsibilities. One pharmacy, for example, uses the title *patient care associate* for all staff members. This title makes the assistants feel like valued members of the team. Kim Swiger emphasizes the importance of training technicians and store staff in their new roles. "They will do a better job and help in marketing services when the opportunity arises over the phone or with customers. It also shows them you value them as team members."

Keep a file of journal articles that highlight the benefits of pharmaceutical care. Use these articles to educate physicians, third-party payers, and other health care providers. These articles will reinforce your position and lend credibility to your efforts.

Finally, don't neglect your own education and training needs. Thoroughly research a disease state before you decide to develop a service around it. Get patient education materials from advocacy groups, such as the American Lung Association or American Diabetes Association. Contact local, state, and national pharmacy associations to find materials. Review major medical and pharmacy journals on your own, or start a journal club with colleagues and staff. Diane Schultz emphasizes the importance of getting trained yourself before you start. "Many pharmacists need and want training, and that is the first step," she notes. She has taken advantage of Washington State Pharmacists Association and other national pharmacy association and pharmaceutical manufacturer professional development training programs.

As you begin to integrate patient-focused care into your practice, you may find it difficult to identify drug-therapy problems. Pharmacists in one location discovered that initially they found about one drug-related problem a day. A year later, with additional experience and education, they find approximately five a day. As Kim Swiger puts it, "Take every opportunity to participate in educational programs whether local, state, or national. It reinforces what you are doing and expands your knowledge base."

Education is paramount for pharmacist Curt Barr, who focuses on empowering patients to take charge of their health. His father was a general practitioner physician and surgeon. Barr says of his father:

He had a very compassionate and caring attitude. I learned his empathetic style of responding to people and copied it when I started empowering my pharmacy patients by educating them to take better care of themselves. I knew I was doing it right when a patient came to me one day and said that without my advice and help he would have died from a medication.

Barr emphasizes patient education, incorporating home visits into his pharmacy practice, teaching home monitoring of glucose, cholesterol, blood pressure, and asthma self-monitoring, among many other services.

Education is central to pharmaceutical care practice. Educate yourself, your staff, your patients, and your community. And be sure to reach out to the physicians as well. They may not understand what you offer initially, and it is important to help them understand just what you are trying to do. Kim Swiger emphasizes the importance of working with physicians. She states, "Physician marketing can be a challenge [but] we have learned that long-term relationship building is effective." When new programs are undertaken, such as Project ImPACT: Osteoporosis, Swiger works to educate the physician community in advance and help build awareness of the positive results such programs can produce. Several family practitioners have been invited to tour the pharmacy and see the services offered first hand. All these gestures have been rewarded by the good will and understanding of their mission the pharmacists have won from physicians.

MANAGING FINANCIAL MATTERS

As you begin integrating patient-focused care into your practice, you will have two major financial issues to consider:

- How to pay for the expenditures needed to provide the new services
- How to arrange payment for the services you offer

At first you may be reluctant to ask your patients to pay for pharmaceutical care services. The focus now, however, is on providing a range of services to improve patient health outcomes. You may argue that you feel uncomfortable charging for services that customers think you have always provided for free. Today's pharmacists are focusing on the total health care of their patients, not just on their medication. Thus, by offering a broader range of services, they have earned the right to be compensated for them.

In 1996 the APhA conducted its National Pharmacy Consumer Survey, which demonstrated patient interest in receiving pharmaceutical care services and a willingness to pay for them. Investigators found that 69% of patients had a "very favorable" or "somewhat favorable" attitude toward the described services. Moreover, almost one third suggested that they were "very likely" or "somewhat likely" to consider switching to those pharmacies that provide pharmaceutical care. This support opens the door to justifying charges for comprehensive care services. The considerable knowledge and expertise pharmacists provide do in fact impact the patients' quality of life.

Receiving payment is only part of the financial picture. In order to provide new services you will need to redesign your pharmacy and will thus incur expenses. Having an accurate financial picture is essential. What financial resources are available and what must be obtained? You also need to determine what current products and services you might be able to eliminate to free up cash and space. You may want to consider securing a loan from a financial institution to pay for modifications to the facility and equipment. While the financial aspects of providing patient-focused care may seem daunting, you can conquer them successfully through careful assessment and planning.

Pharmacist Laurie Kaup's experience is a good model for those interested in moving into pharmaceutical care. She began her career in an entrepreneurial way. She first secured a business loan. "To open our pharmacy," she relates, "my husband and I borrowed $45,000 from a local businessman. He was a local insurance agent, but he had faith in us and taught us what servicing the customer was all about, as well as what life in a small town would be like." Further, Kaup adds, "If we had not been able to make a business plan with 5-year projections per the instructions of our pharmacy administration professor, Ronaldo Brusadin, now with the Nevada College of Pharmacy, I am sure we would not have gotten the loan."

In her pharmaceutical care practice, documentation is done for services, so patients can take a copy of the pharmacists' notes to their physician. Charges for services vary, but they bill patients using an 80/20 rule. If the patient has insurance, they pay 20% out of pocket and the insurer gets a bill for the remaining 80%. Where appropriate, they use the HCFA 1500 forms for billing. "Since we are JCAHO [Joint Commission on the Accreditation of Healthcare Organizations] accredited," Kaup says proudly, "we have a quality improvement committee that meets regularly, comprised of patients and physicians who provide feedback on how we are doing."

Tina Lampe-Izaguirre and her colleagues have received strong support from their company in billing and payment matters. In addition to the patient base built through detailing, Eckerd provides corporate support in generating contracts for services with HMOs and employer groups. Fees and billing for services is determined corporately with 80 to 85% of payments from third parties. The center transmits billing information using HCFA 1500 forms to Eckerd's corporate managed care group on a biweekly basis. Charges are based on the Medicare RBVRS — the same one that physicians use.

Here is one more success story in implementing new patient services and getting paid for them. In 1997 Diane Shultz initiated an innovative practice in emergency contraception services at Drug Emporium. She and her colleagues worked with physicians to create collaborative practice arrangements with prescriptive authority. Diane was able to secure a grant to fund program marketing and in the first year alone 3500 patients were seen in 18 of 24 stores where the services were offered. They charge patients $35 for the service and treat it like a prescription, moving it efficiently from a workflow standpoint. It takes about 10 minutes to counsel the patients; payment comes from cash, Medicaid, and pharmacies using HCFA 1500 forms. Pharmaceutical care is working out for Diane Shultz professionally and financially.

Whether you practice independently, as part of a group, or within a corporate structure, your professional services are valuable to your patients. If pharmacists reach out to patients, their physicians, each other, and to the communities they serve documenting care plans, they would find patients will come to depend on them. This will result in professional satisfaction — both financial and spiritual — similar to that experienced by the pharmacists profiled in the next section of this book. These people pioneered a new model of care with courage and commitment to community service. They found it brought them professional satisfaction and rewards that were previously unattainable.

REFERENCES

1. TheAPhA/NWDA Concept Pharmacy Project, American Pharmaceutical Association and the National Wholesale Druggists Association, Reston, VA, 1997 (now available from the Healthcare Distributors and Manufacturers Association, Reston, VA).
2. Klotz, R.S., Pharmacist-physician link: Keys to effective outcomes management, Monograph 15, in *Value Added Services* series, Engle, J.P., ed., APhA, Washington, D.C., 1995
2. Tomechko, M. et al., Q and A from the pharmaceutical care project in Minnesota, *Am. Pharm.*, April 1995, NS35, 4, 30–38.

4

LEADERSHIP AND SUCCESS: LESSONS FROM NONPHARMACISTS

Go the extra mile. It's never crowded.

—Executive Speedwriter Newsletter

If one advances confidently in the direction of his dreams, and endeavors to live the life which he has imagined, he will meet with a success unexpected in common hours.

—Henry David Thoreau

When setting out to discover if pharmacist innovators are different, we began by looking at what others had found different about those whom they labeled innovators, leaders, or successes. Then, having some insight into their habits, behaviors, beliefs, and values, we began to interview more than 50 pharmacy innovators to assess whether or not they shared some of these same characteristics that led people in other professions or industries to find success. Here is what we learned about success and leadership.

WHAT IS SUCCESS?

Poets, philosophers, writers, and storytellers have made whole books, treatises, and manuscripts reflecting upon the meaning of success. Yet the *Oxford American Dictionary* defines it simply as "a favorable outcome, doing what was desired or attempted, the attainment of wealth or fame or position."[1] Using as our reference this respected dictionary, we argue that obtaining wealth, fame, or position in relationship to success is really an outcome of having done that which was desired or attempted. If so, then the real essence of success comes from doing what one wants and doing it toward a good end. In support of this, Kouzes and Posner state very simply, that regardless of the scope of a person's influence, "success is leaving the area a better place than when you found it."[2] Blanchard and Bowles write that success is individual, that each person harbors different hopes, dreams, and desires for his or her life.[3]

> To be successful, the first thing to do is fall in love with your work.
>
> —Sister Mary Lauretta

In his new book, *The American Dream: Stories from the Heart of Our Nation*, Dan Rather describes success as achieving the American dream. He writes there is no typical American dream; that for some, the dream is freedom, for others, fortune, family, or service to one's fellows. For others, success comes from the great emphasis placed on the pursuit of happiness or keeping the innovative spirit alive. "Regardless of how we define it," Rather says, "the American dream defines us as a people."[4]

Tim Tweedie writes on what it means to succeed by stating:

> Most people see success as being rich and famous or powerful and influential. Others see it as being at the top of their profession and standing out from the rest. The wise see success in a more personal way; they see it as achieving the goals they have set for themselves, and then feeling pride and satisfaction in their accomplishments. True success is felt in the heart, not measured by money and power. So be true to yourself and achieve the goals you set, for success is reaching those goals and feeling proud of what you have accomplished.[5]

The heroes you will meet in this book — much like Tom Brokaw's ordinary people doing extraordinary things for the greater good cited on page 3 — have all achieved success. Each is doing what he or she wants toward a good end, leaving things better in the areas they touch than they found them. But does being successful make one a leader?

WHAT IS LEADERSHIP AND ARE LEADERS SUCCESSFUL?

When one thinks of leaders, very often famous people who have influenced great numbers of individuals, communities, or countries come to mind, such as presidents, war heroes, activists, sports figures, and entertainers, among others. Yet, leadership also can be applied to those who have achieved much smaller victories. Is the person who helps an elderly individual cross a street a leader? What about those who set good examples by always finding good in others? Are innovative pharmacists being leaders when they help a patient with health plan issues or medication problems?

Stephen Covey argues in *The 7 Habits of Highly Effective People* that interpersonal leadership is a necessary ingredient for being able to work with others in a win–win fashion.[6] Indeed, he defines a leader as one whose example is followed, who takes the lead, influencing and guiding the actions of others. For some, the notion of them being in a leadership role is intimidating while for others it is a natural extension of moving forward with what they want to do. How then, do you get to be a leader?

> To become a leader, you must become yourself; become the maker of your own life.
>
> —Warren Bennis

Warren Bennis has a long career studying leadership — both what it is and how people become leaders. In his second book, *On Becoming a Leader*, Bennis notes that "leaders are people who express themselves fully. They know who they are, what their strengths and weaknesses are, how to fully deploy their strengths and compensate for their weaknesses. They also know what they want, why they want it, and how to communicate what they want to others in order to gain their cooperation and support."[7] Finally, Bennis says, "They know how to achieve their goals. No leader sets out to be a leader, rather, people set out to live their lives, expressing themselves fully. When that expression is of value, they become leaders." He further notes, "the point is not to become a leader. The point is to become yourself, to use yourself completely — all your skills, gifts and energies — in order to make your vision manifest."

While interpersonal leadership is important in working with others and in implementing what you want to do, becoming a leader is often a by-product of success — doing what you want to do toward a good end.

WHAT KIND OF PEOPLE BECOME LEADERS?

What characteristics or traits do leaders exhibit? Are they loud or quiet? Are they controlling or giving? Are they in charge of large or small companies? Are they involved in activities outside their work? The answer is that leaders come in every size, shape, and from every place, but do they share common traits that help identify them as leaders?

Bennis makes a strong case that leaders are made, not born, and are made more by being themselves than by any external means. As they set out to accomplish their goals they get farther by expressing themselves with behavior that defines them as leaders. And they continue to grow and develop all their lives. The most pivotal characteristic of a leader, Bennis believes, is their concern with a guiding purpose or overarching vision and the discipline and perseverance in their quest to implement it.

> Yes, you can be a dreamer and doer too, if you will remove one word from your vocabulary, impossible.
>
> —H. Robert Schuller

In his interviews with nearly 30 leaders from various industries, characteristics of leadership revealed to Bennis were:

1. Guiding vision. A leader has a clear idea of what he or she wants to do personally and professionally and the strength to pursue it in spite of setbacks and failures. Unless you know where you are going, how can you get there?
2. Passion for the "promises of life," but more importantly for a specific vocation, profession, or course of action.
3. Integrity, comprised of self-knowledge, candor (honesty of thought and action, devotion to principle), and maturity (learning to lead by following, learning to be dedicated, observant, and capable of working with and learning from others, never servile, always truthful). Integrity is also the basis of trust — a characteristic that is earned and needed to get people to help you accomplish your goals.
4. Curiosity and daring. Leaders want to learn and take risks. They embrace errors and learn from them and from adversity.

There are no shortcuts to anyplace worth going.

—Beverly Sills

Much of the Bennis work on leaders parallels that of Stephen Covey who worked to identify the habits of highly effective people, i.e., having a vision, being proactive, prioritizing, gaining trust, and working with people so all can achieve more together than any could achieve individually. In his book, *The 7 Habits of Highly Effective People*, he says there are seven behaviors that identify people who think and act differently from the norm. Yet, in the pharmaceutical literature, if one were to ask, are pharmaceutical care innovators acting and thinking differently from the norm? The literature is silent. Covey writes that the behaviors of effective people are powerful lessons that others can use to motivate personal change.[1] For pharmacists then, these lessons have significant application for anyone contemplating or implementing a venture into professional growth and adopting a new care paradigm. These habits and their relevance are:

1. Be proactive. Use the four fundamental human endowments (self-awareness, imagination, conscience, and independent will) to choose your behavior. Realize that behavior is a function of decisions not conditions. Thus, practicing an advanced level of pharmaceutical care should be made as a matter of personal choice not as an edict from a professional guru or group.
2. Begin with the end in mind. All things are created twice, first in the mind and then in reality, and success comes from having a clear plan of what you want to achieve. Thus, for pharmacists, the ability to envision pharmaceutical care and place it in context with their ethical values and guidelines is paramount in achieving success. It also means that those who write guidelines for pharmaceutical care introduced as the mainstream tenet of the profession will have a hard time gaining acceptance until such time as individual pharmacists can see it in their mind's eye and apply a word picture acceptable to their personal frame of professional behavior.
3. Put first things first. This is the exercise of free will that makes effective self-management possible. For pharmacists, it applies to those who are disciplined, act with strength of purpose, and organize and execute around priorities. Thus, pharmaceutical care will not be mainstream until pharmacists make a personal effort at setting it as a professional and personal priority.

4. Think win–win. This means being able to go beyond reciting the golden rule and acting on it. For many, workplace problems are seen as coming from the people they must deal with rather than coming from the paradigm they must work under. Thus for pharmaceutical care to work, it must be applied with fairness to all patients.

5. Seek first to understand, then to be understood. Communication (reading, writing, speaking, and listening) is an essential skill for anyone to be effective and successful in life, and without this ability any pharmacist dedicated to pharmaceutical care will find success a difficult pathway.

6. Synergize. Synergy is the essence of principle-centered leadership. It takes the four unique human endowments, the skills of empathetic communication, and the motivation behind a win–win attitude so that relationships can be built to produce an outcome greater than its parts. Thus, to the pharmacist wanting to provide an advanced level of practice, he or she must first build a level of creative cooperation so patients see this new environment of care fulfilling to both.

7. Renewal. Preserving, enhancing, and renewing the four dimensions (physical, mental, social/emotional, and spiritual) of one's nature in a wise and balanced way preserves and enhances one's ability to do work. Pharmacists who miss out on this balancing act as a long-term way of life will not have what it takes to make an effective commitment to a new paradigm of care.

Pharmacy is a health profession that talks about its members as being part of the health care team. Yet, in reviewing the pharmacy literature about innovative and visionary pharmacy practice, there is little help for achieving community-based pharmacists as accepted members of the health team. However, in the business literature, the meaning of teamwork is illustrated as having four key ingredients. Ken Blanchard and Sheldon Bowles write that the magic of working together exists when there is:

- Worthwhile work providing purpose and value
- Empowerment that enables one to unleash and develop skills, relationships, and communication
- Flexibility to create team power and optimal performance
- Recognition and appreciation to keep an accent on the positive and morale high[7]

The premise behind Blanchard and Bowles' four key ingredients is that none of us is as smart as all of us. Traditionalists in pharmacy would do well to search out innovators and listen to their stories, for it is their collective wisdom that will enable the profession to turn itself around and embark on a new journey in providing enhanced professional service. It will be those rugged individuals who, through patient–pharmacist encounters, hard work, perseverance, willingness to change, and passion to conduct the business of their profession in new and exciting ways, will give life to new professional paradigms.

Sharing their dreams, stories, and successes, they will open new pathways for others to follow. In fact, they will likely have had as much failure along their journey as they have had success. For example, there is a favorite story about an American who failed and, finally, succeeded. But it is also a story about a man who exemplified hard work, mastered persistence, changed himself, conducted business in new and exciting ways and had to contend with many obstacles on a career path that eventually led him to higher levels of service:

At 21, his first business failed.
At 23, he ran for a state political office and lost.
At 24, his second business failed.
At 27, he suffered a nervous breakdown.
At 29, he ran for the U.S. Congress and lost.
At 31, he ran for Congress a second time and lost.
At 37, he ran for Congress a third time and won.
At 46, he ran for vice president and lost.
At 49, he ran for the U.S. Senate and lost.
Then, at the age of 51, he ran for the U.S. presidency and won.

This individual, who was persistent, patient, and sought a higher level of service for himself and his country, was Abraham Lincoln, the 16th U.S. president, and the only president that ever had to face the potential split of the union.

> Failure is sometimes the raw material God uses to make us be successful again.
>
> —Anon.

To bring pharmaceutical care into communities, many pharmacists are going to have to change. Change is difficult. Most people resist change, especially if they feel loss of status, income, job security, or prestige will result.[8] So rather than promoting pharmaceutical care as a role change, pharmacy leadership may find less resistance in community settings once a few pharmacists adopt it as an entrepreneurial challenge, are successful, and are willing to talk to others about their success. According to author and business researcher James R. Cook, entrepreneurs pioneer ventures where risk is high, and where creativity, persistence, and inevitable success make that person a leader and contemporary hero.[9] Now that pharmacy has been buffeted by the cold chill of managed care and other market forces, it is even more important to recognize that pharmaceutical care can be initiated if rugged and beleaguered individuals are willing to risk putting it into action. To a great extent, the profession's future and economic well-being will depend on exactly the type of people whom we interviewed — leaders and contemporary heroes.

> In a world where there is so much to be done, I felt strongly impressed that there must be something for me to do.
>
> —Dorothea Dix

HEROES AS LEADERS: COMMON ATTRIBUTES

Armed with some new ideas about pharmaceutical care, success, and leadership, we interviewed men and women making significant contributions to patient care in community settings. We selected 15 in all for this book, but talked to three times as many. Our interviews reinforced what we suspected. Pharmacist trailblazers:

- Share a common set of attributes even though they practice in different regions and with different types of patients
- Had very different personal pathways to get to where they are today
- Exhibit the confidence to take decisive action with boldness and determination

We believe pharmacist trailblazers are motivated and determined people who realize that nothing will be accomplished until responsible action is taken. In our interviews, we tried to find out how this action was demonstrated by asking for examples of situations where they:

- Refused to admit defeat
- Finished what they started
- Stayed self-motivated for long periods

- Committed to a plan to accomplish a specific objective
- Found creative ways around obstacles
- Had to go it alone

Taking responsible action arises from a desire to act in a certain manner where the incentive is either internal (i.e., a search for praise or acceptance) or external (i.e., a desire for rewards such as money), and these factors become the stimuli or motivators for professional satisfaction and success. The psychologist Abraham Maslow wrote that people are moved to action in order to satisfy a hierarchical series of needs. Beginning at the bottom, the hierarchy moves through physiological needs (food, air, and water), on to safety needs (clothing, shelter), followed by the needs for belonging, love, esteem, and self-actualization. Each person has a set of these motivating factors and each person feels them and feeds them differently at various times and under various conditions. Maslow also believed that fewer than 50% of all people realize their need for self-actualization and often get bogged down meeting needs lower on the hierarchy.

A second source of a pharmacist trailblazer's ability to take responsible action is boldness. These people are willing to take risks without knowing what the rewards will be ahead of time, challenge the status quo, keep their integrity intact, and keep their emotions steady while facing uncertainty. Acting boldly appears to be an outcome of how people deal with their fears, such as fear of disapproval, the unknown, taking a risk, and failure.

Boldness occurs when passion rises and vanity falls.

—Kevin McCarthy

The third source of a pharmacist's ability to take responsible action is self-confidence. Pharmacists exude confidence when they do not let past mistakes erode their self-worth, let fear stop them from running against the grain, or hold back on what they believe is intuitively right. The genesis of the word *confidence* comes from the Latin *confidere*, to trust in someone. We believe the pharmacist who behaves as a trailblazer places a lot of trust in someone, and that person is himself or herself.

If you have not often felt the joy of doing a kind act, you have neglected much, and most of all yourself.

—A. Nielsen

Other attributes shared by the pharmacists you'll read about are:

A passion for patients — the overarching passion that drives them is getting up every day and working in a profession where they help people. Fundamentally, helping people is a key part of their fulfillment.

Know thyself — in order to find happiness as pharmacists in the practice setting they chose, they have a clear understanding of what they want, what they are good at, what they do not like, what they find limiting, and how they want to be treated.

The gap between today and tomorrow — knowing their passion and themselves, they can assess if there is a gap between where they are in the profession today and where they want to be tomorrow.

The courage to act — being able to assess this gap allows them to create specific plans to move forward if they are at a place different from where they want to be. As Bennis says, the first step toward change is to refuse to be deployed by others and to choose to deploy yourself.

Collaborating vs. competing — they have what Covey calls the "attitude of abundance," the belief that there is enough for everyone and the best way to get it is to collaborate with others rather than by competing.

Patience and persistence — all have suffered setbacks and found it took more time to achieve their goals than they had planned. As a result, they learned to be persistent, not to give up, and to continue pursuing their goals while enjoying the smaller victories toward the end.

Sharing support — all point to the network of colleagues, family, and friends that provides their support, sharing information and helping each other. Time and time again, they point to this shared support system as a key resource, often formed through their participation in professional organizations.

The really happy [person] is one who can enjoy the scenery on a detour.

—Anon.

REFERENCES

1. Erlich, R. et al., *Oxford American Dictionary*, Avon Books, New York, 1980.
2. Kouzes, J.M. and Pozner, B.Z., *Credibility*, Josey-Bass Publishers, San Francisco, 1993.
3. Blanchard, K. and Bowles, S., *High Five: The Magic of Working Together*, HarperCollins Publishers, New York, 2001.
4. Rather, D., *The American Dream: Stories from the Heart of Our Nation*, William Morrow & Co., New York, 2001.
5. Tweedie, T., *The Language of Success*, Blue Mountain Press, Boulder, CO, 1999.
6. Covey, S.R., *The 7 Habits of Highly Effective People*, Simon & Schuster, New York, 1989.
7. Bennis, W., *On Becoming a Leader*, Addison-Wesley, New York, 1989.
8. Kirkpatrick, D.L., *How to Manage Change Effectively*, Jossey Bass Publishers, San Francisco, 1986, p. 34.
9. Cook, J.R., *The Start-Up Entrepreneur*, Harper & Row, New York, 1986.

II

UNCOMMON PEOPLE

ACKNOWLEDGMENTS

The authors gratefully acknowledge the time given by the following pharmacists as we intruded into their busy professional and personal lives. We appreciate their gracious and candid manner, and their introspection as they explained to us how they became peak performers and innovators in pharmacy. We found them passionate, undaunted, and mentally and physically fit. Their approach to pharmaceutical care is to bring to it a positive attitude and a belief that a profession's challenges can be overcome by persistence. These special pharmacists are:

Chapter 5	Marla Ahlgrimm, R.Ph., Women's Health America, Madison, WI
Chapter 6	Curt Barr, Pharm.D., Blair Pharmacy, Blair, NE
Chapter 7	Eric Graf, R.Ph., Ritzman's Pharmacy, Wadsworth, OH
Chapter 8	Judith Sommers-Hanson, R.Ph., Dominick's Pharmacies, Buffalo Grove, IL
Chapter 9	Kelley Hofer, R.Ph., Southwest Medical Center, Camas, WA
Chapter 10	Laurie Kaup, R.Ph., Kaup Pharmacy, Fort Recovery, OH
Chapter 11	Rick Mohall, Pharm.D., Eckerd Patient Care Center, Clearwater, FL
Chapter 12	Max Peoples, R.Ph., Uptown Pharmacy, Westerville, OH
Chapter 13	Beverly Schaefer, R.Ph., Katterman's Pharmacy, Seattle, WA
Chapter 14	Diane Schultz, Pharm.D., Pharmaceutical Care Coordinator, Long's Drug Stores, Seattle, WA
Chapter 15	Michelle Shibley, Pharm.D., Richmond Apothecaries, Richmond, VA
Chapter 16	Kim Swiger, R.Ph., Ukrop's Supermarket & Pharmacy, Richmond, VA
Chapter 17	Greg Wedin, R.Ph., formerly of Wedin Drug, Glencoe, MN

5

MARLA AHLGRIMM: TEACHING HEALTH AND WELLNESS

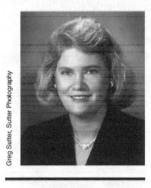

Greg Sutter, Sutter Photography

Marla Ahlgrimm

With a national patient base reaching hundreds of thousands of people, primarily women, Marla Ahlgrimm has taken her vision of pharmacy practice and created a truly one-of-a-kind practice, one that is helping people learn health and wellness practices that will last a lifetime. She attributes her practice's beginnings to a series of coincidences that led to the creation of a women's health pharmacy with emphasis on holistic care and compounded natural hormone replacement therapy. The recognition of and ability to take these events and learn from them and then apply that knowledge to move forward are a key to her success.

For example, in his critically acclaimed book, *The Celestine Prophecy*,[1] author James Redfield uses the tale of a lost Peruvian manuscript to teach readers important insights about their lives. The first is related to coincidences that occur. We know they are real, but don't understand their meaning until years later. The basic message is that everything in life happens for a reason — that there really are no coincidences. As one of the main characters says, "The first insight is a reconsideration of the inherent mystery that surrounds our individual lives on this planet. We are experiencing these mysterious coincidences…. We are sensing again, as in childhood, that there is another side of life that we have yet to discover, some other process operating behind the scenes."

In Ahlgrimm's case, she was trying to help someone overcome suffering. In the late 1970s, during her time as a student at the University of Wisconsin, she worked at a pharmacy. The wife of the pharmacy's owner was severely affected by mood swings 2 weeks each month and had been prescribed Valium and amphetamines, which were not relieving the symptoms. The woman ran across an article describing another woman, who had just moved to Madison from New York, who had similar issues and was receiving treatment in Europe. As Ahlgrimm recalls, "It was the ultimate story of patient frustration with traditional medical practice not listening to the real problem, but reacting in a way that says, 'You're a woman, therefore it must all be in your head,' and treating it accordingly."

They did detailed library research on the European ideas and began to incorporate them into a treatment program relying on natural progesterone. "It was if a cloud had lifted for her after a short time on the hormones," recalls Ahlgrimm. They began compounding natural hormones for other patients. Soon, other doctors began referring women there and word spread that the pharmacy was teaching people to manage their menstrual and hormonal cycle history — which they coined premenstrual syndrome (PMS). Within 2 years the pharmacy ended up with 500 patients. She reflects, "We talked to people about their health vs. just dispensing prescriptions. That was a hard concept for some people, including the owner's father who wondered what on earth we were thinking. It was apparent if we wanted to continue, we would have to go it on our own. So my preceptor, his wife and I left. Here was the practice I had envisioned in school, it was right in front of us, we were doing it and we wanted to keep on and expand it."

EXPANDING THE PRACTICE

She was only 26 years old and had no idea what challenges she would face because of her gender and age. There were issues about finding someone willing to rent her space. When a 700-sq. ft. office was found for the pharmacy, the State Board of Pharmacy struggled with licensing it because of the unique nature of its practice. Finally, the media picked up on the story and, once again, barriers came down, word spread, and within 18 months the pharmacy moved to a 5000-sq. ft. space with a staff of nine.

Recently, her Madison-based practice moved into its fourth location, comprising 17,000 sq. ft with 35 employees serving 10,000 physicians and hundreds of thousands of patients. She has written several books and newsletters, has appeared on national and local television, and has become a minor celebrity in the Madison area.

LOYAL PATIENTS

"Our patients never leave and many have been with us for more than 20 years." She attributes that to their specialized yet individual approach to care. Everything they do is based on natural hormone replacement that cannot be patented, a fact she believes has led the traditional pharmaceutical industry to miss the mark in treatment in spite of their commitment to research. The practice focuses on exercise, nutrition, and lifestyle management offering a continuum of care.

One program is called Restore. It is a comprehensive holistic program prescribed by many referring physicians. In the program, levels of five baseline hormones are measured using a test researched and developed by Ahlgrimm. The test is saliva based and costs between $30 and $40. If therapy is needed, which is the case about 35% of the time, it is customized for the patient over a 2- to 3-month period. The initial patient visit lasts about an hour and is scheduled following at least a 4- to 6-hour work-up. The software used to manage patients was also self-created and detailed medical histories are documented. The complete Restore program is $295.

What may be surprising to some is that Ahlgrimm says about 65% of the patients she sees need only self-management. You might wonder how the practice supports itself? About half its revenues are derived from product sales and the other half from books, newsletters, and other informational materials that can help educate people to self-manage their conditions. Ahlgrimm recognizes how advanced the ideas and program are and, as a result, does not slow her or the practice's progress by trying to get insurers to pay. She believes there is just too much else on which to focus and has found a way to support the practice without direct insurance payment. "When you are focused on wellness creation rather than disease management, the health care infrastructure in this country just can't handle it and doesn't know how to process it. Maybe someday it will catch up to us," she notes.

RUNNING OUT OF TIME

Her greatest fear in life — "I'm going to run out of time to do all the things I want to" — is also reflected in her practice. At age 45, her present challenge is creating the plan for where she wants to be at 50 and how she is going to get there. It is a constant evolution. "My staff is great. They really want to help me implement ideas. But, at times, they have to put the brakes on me — as they like to say, 'The idea department is closed.'" The 35-member team is comprised of five pharmacists, four technicians, four health educators, three nurses, and the remainder in the customer service/order entry department, which handles up to 1000 calls a day. The practice compounds about 400 prescriptions each day as well. She also relies on medical writers in Los Angeles, a business/sales consultant in Atlanta, and a research alliance in Germany.

Appropriately, the new practice is on Deming Drive — named after quality guru Edward Deming. It is called the Women's Health America Building and is Ahlgrimm's worldwide headquarters. It houses areas for dispensing, nurse and case management, laboratory, compounding, and counseling. It is in the heart of the biotechnology area of Madison. She hopes to teach the 14 Deming principles of quality improvement there.

Typical of her support of the local community, local artists were commissioned to create the artwork that adorns the building. This urban, entrepreneurial center has a network of support for innovation that is well funded by the state and supported by the governor.

A FAMILY OF ENTREPRENEURS

It is not difficult to see where Ahlgrimm gets her entrepreneurial talent. It was part of her family history and has been refined by the Madison environment. "My father was in explosives engineering applied to road construction. He was only 1 of 50 people with the specialized knowledge base in the country. We moved a lot, and when he tired of it, we settled here and he began teaching at the University." Her mother is a home economics teacher and her two younger brothers run a company that she started. Her stints as a Mineral Point tour guide and in sales also fueled the fire. She described Madison as a city "where possibilities are all around you."

While no single individual influenced her more than others, she credits some of her vision to reading about Eugene White's office-based practice in *Remington's Practice of Pharmacy*[2] during school. "I remember thinking [that] I can do that" she says. "It showed me what practice could become rather than what it was. I saw the positive side and wanted to build it."

She has a creative side that is unusually developed among those with scientific education and training. "I liked the creative classes in junior and senior high school — art and music. I started college as a music major playing piano and trumpet. I was very intense, serious, and liked everything. But I didn't want to be a starving artist," she notes. "I also liked chemistry and biology. It was a high school guidance counselor who mentioned pharmacy to me one day walking home from school. He pointed out that it combined people, science, business, research, and teaching. That was it for me." She believes it is important to know yourself well enough to make a good career match. Her mom taught science after home economics and Ahlgrimm credits that to stoking her interest.

That said, her mother's influence didn't go far enough, according to her. "The most humiliating thing I ever have tried is learning to cook. Mom tried. When I built my first house and moved in, it was 6 months before I learned the stove didn't work because I hadn't turned it on!" That anecdote is typical of her sense of humor. One can appreciate her ability to be self-deprecating, as well as her strengths. She identifies most with the labels of innovator, teacher, professional, motivator, visionary, and optimist.

But in spite of that optimism, the thing that worries her most is the regulator's inability to keep pace with innovative practices. "There is a lot of overregulation and misunderstanding by regulators and I think it can be a frustrating waste of time, energy and money to educate them. And yet that is important if we want to be able to allow the growth of ideas and make pharmacy more collaborative."

She is one who loves work so much, she actually is sad to leave for the weekends. But, she fills her time with her terriers — an Airedale and two Westies. "They are so bright and fun to be with. They think on their feet. They are bold and stout of heart as a breed," she says. She also likes golf and appreciates adventure travel. "I like to take 3 weeks off each year and immerse myself in a holistic, adventure travel experience." She hopes to spend time with the Hill tribes of Cambodia and venture to Ethiopia as well. She finds such trips help open her eyes to cultures that are more quality-of-life focused with integrated structures of family, friends, and support.

What is next for Ahlgrimm? She is rolling out the Restore program worldwide, is creating a men's Restore program with a type II diabetes focus, and hopes to implement comprehensive drug therapy monitoring services. It will require major investment and she is looking at funding sources. She wants to build a business that can support the employees living "happily ever after" in the spirit of a true optimist.

That giving spirit will likely be rewarded in the way she hopes people remember her: "as a role model and innovator who makes things look easy and who recognizes the potential of people and situations."

ADVICE TO OTHERS

■ Don't accept the way things are always done. Create and innovate.
■ If you think you are wrong, move on from where you are. Push the limits of your experience, ideas, and pursue new ways of thinking.
■ Put yourself in new and challenging situations. It is how you grow.
■ Take responsibility for your own happiness and ask yourself when you go to your practice, "Why am I here today?" For me, the answer is "I'm here to make a difference."
■ "Sometimes when you reach a roadblock, you just have to put some things on a back burner until society catches up to you."
■ Be an internal optimist. Ask yourself, "What is the worst thing that can happen?"
■ "Be secure with change. If you live in self-doubt without positive role models, you might as well hang it up."

REFERENCES

1. Redfield, J., *The Celestine Prophecy*, Warner Books, New York, 1993.
2. Gennaro, A.R., ed., *Remington: The Science and Practice of Pharmacy*, Lippincott, Williams & Wilkins, Philadelphia.

6

CURT BARR: APPLYING THE MEDICAL MODEL TO PHARMACY PRACTICE

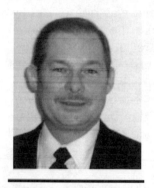

Curt Barr

Curt Barr comes from a family of health professionals. His father, uncle, cousin, and grandfather were physicians, and other family members chose fields such as nursing. Barr learned from his family what it means to be of service to others. "Being in such a giving family," he recalls, "I learned at an early age what would become my vision ... of what health care was all about by seeing it up close and personal ... especially in a small Nebraska town of under a thousand, where everybody knew who you were and set expected behavior." Barr remembers that his initial desire to help people came from watching his father take care of his patients. He was a general practitioner physician and surgeon with a compassionate and caring attitude. Barr learned his empathic style of responding to people by emulating his father. "I started empowering my pharmacy patients by educating them to take better care of themselves. I knew I was doing it right when a patient came to me one day and said that without my advice and help he would have died from a medication."

HOW CURT BARR DEVELOPED A PASSION FOR PHARMACY

Curt Barr earned a B.S. in biology from Wayne State University in Nebraska and upon graduation was offered a job in a laboratory in Omaha. After a year of exemplary work he was asked to transfer to a new facility in Kansas City. He turned the offer down because he wanted to follow in his father's and grandfather's footsteps and be a physician. He applied to medical school, but was not accepted at the University of Nebraska Medical School or Creighton University Medical School. Instead, the admissions officials at Creighton University Pharmacy School wrote him a letter stating they would be interested in having him in their program. Upon the urging and advice of his wife Vicki, Barr accepted their offer. A month into pharmacy school, his professor told him to read in *Remington's Practice of Pharmacy*[1] about the office-practice pharmacy of Eugene White of Virginia. He was hooked. "From reading about what Eugene White was doing, I knew from that day forward I was committed to make the medical model of health care work in pharmacy practice," he recalls. "This is why I opened my first pharmacy in a culturally diverse neighborhood of Omaha three weeks after I graduated from pharmacy school."

Barr's first pharmacy was in a diverse neighborhood with many Medicaid patients. A few years later he purchased a pharmacy in Blair, a suburb on the north side of Omaha, where he thought he would like to raise his family. He was gratified when several dozen patients from his first site followed him.

Later, at an APhA meeting, Barr says, "I got to meet Virginia pharmacist Carl Emswiller and my other professional hero, Eugene White. They both became friends and mentors giving support and encouragement. Additional encouragement came from my friend E. Richard Coe of Phoenix and [from] all three I got a lot of 'attaboys,' 'you should go for it,' 'you can do it,' and 'never forget people will come to you knowing what they want, it's your job to give them what they need.'"

When Barr took over an established pharmacy his unorthodox style was soon the talk of the town. For instance, before he would dispense high blood pressure medicines he would first take the patient's blood pressure and record that reading in a specially designed patient record. Patients were happy, but physicians were upset. He won their approval, however, when he showed them the inaccuracies of having patients take their own blood pressure on a machine about to be installed in a local bank. Physicians quickly accepted that Barr was both an advocate for doctors and their patients. His practice has been on a growth curve ever since. Today, when you visit Barr Pharmacy, Curt Barr and his staff of 14 people (including one full-time and two part-time pharmacists) are filling about 110 prescriptions per day, but they are also providing pharmaceutical care services such as:

- Teaching blood glucose self-monitoring to diabetics
- Teaching self-monitoring of asthma triggers
- Teaching self-monitoring of blood pressure to hypertensive patients
- Teaching self-monitoring of cholesterol levels
- Teaching self-monitoring of INR levels for patients on anticoagulation therapy
- Providing nicotine cessation programs
- Providing pharmacist home visits for:
    Monitoring drug dating
    Medication compliance support and organization of regimens
    Identification of drug therapy problems
- Counseling on side effects, use, purposes of all prescription and nonprescription medications
- Offering in-depth disease management and consultation with parents and guardians
- Offering physician interventions and consultations
- Consulting on formulary changes, DUR, insurance changes
- Offering pharmacy care interventions
- Repackaging medications into unit of use dosing kits
- Resolving prescription and nonprescription drug conflicts
- Providing disease management interventions

Curt Barr believes that it is his job to help every patient take an active role in his or her own health care and that patients should show evidence of that active role by paying him for his services. "I charge $2 per minute or $120 per hour," says Barr, "and no one balks at it on an FFS [fee for service] basis." He adds, "If 80 to 90% of drug costs are covered by insurance there certainly is the ability for a patient to pay me for making sure the drug is taken properly or for me to eliminate a problem that would render a drug ineffective." Barr makes sure that all interventions are documented in hard copy charts so they can be tracked and that all staff are well versed in his credo that they "Take the extra step, be responsible for each patient's therapeutic outcome." Today, approximately 20 patients are seen every day at Barr Pharmacy.

Barr is also proud to point out that another of his philosophical commitments was engrained because of a high school job in a pharmacy. Blackstone Pharmacy in Omaha was run by a husband and wife team, Chuck and Arlene Hoffman. They taught him never to say never to a customer. Further they admonished him to remember that, although as a professional he may leave the office behind, he is never to leave the patient behind. "For example," Barr relates, "one day in Blair Pharmacy a patient came in and commented that she had been diagnosed with COPD [chronic obstructive pulmonary disease] and would soon need an oxygen concentrator. She stated she would like me to get one for her because she trusted me. Soon thereafter I was in the oxygen business." He hired a full-time nurse to handle that new line of business.

Does he ever leave the office behind? When asked, Barr replies, "My wife and I have raised three sons and one is going through Creighton Pharmacy School now. We are very proud of our family and how well they have turned out. My hobbies are the restoration of antique cars and motorcycles. I also enjoy hunting, cooking, and scuba diving. We have enjoyed a lot of family vacations and most of them have been at pharmacy association conventions. I have been very active over the years in my local and state societies as well as APhA and NCPA and credit this for many friendships and talks with innovative pharmacists who have given me more ideas than those I created myself. One honor I do remember well was being named the first Syntex Preceptor of the Year and being elected to serve on the Nebraska Board of Pharmacy. Now, I am looking forward to influencing students through my faculty appointment at Creighton, because if they adopt my medical model for pharmacy practice they can influence positively the therapeutic management of greater numbers of patients than the 7000 that reside in Blair, Nebraska."

ADVICE TO OTHERS

- Start slow — Pick one disease area and try it. It is similar to dosing a geriatric patient using the philosophy of "start low and go slow." So pick out a patient, focus on the patient's need, and follow that patient's need home.
- If you concentrate on taking care of patients, payment takes care of itself. If you worry about what the competition is doing, you will find you are *only* worrying about the competition.

- Strong beliefs to move forward to take care of your fellow man come from a deep feeling within. When you release that feeling into action you will find the response is contagious. When you do a little bit for a lot of people rewards will come in many ways — sometimes only as a smile but a reward nonetheless. These rewards build confidence in what you are doing and keep you going.
- Your attitude matters. You are a professional 24/7/365 for a lot of years, and that will never let you leave a patient behind.
- Better decisions are made by those who understand the larger environment of health care and pharmacy. They are involved in policy making and professional associations. Get involved with your time, talents, and finances and you will be better off for it.
- A Ralph Waldo Emerson piece is printed on every document that I give to students. It reflects my philosophy of what I term *success as a professional*. When all pharmacists understand this philosophy, they too will know success resides in the pharmacist who has found a niche by helping people make the best use of their medications.

REFERENCE

1. Gennaro, A.R., ed., *Remington: The Science and Practice of Pharmacy*, Lippincott, Williams & Wilkins, Philadelphia.

7

ERIC GRAF: THE JOY IN TEACHING OTHERS

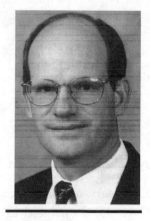

Eric Graf

The Ritzman's chain operates eight pharmacies mostly in small farming communities in northeastern Ohio. In 1997 the owners began converting all of their pharmacies into the area's best resource on natural health products. Because of Eric Graf, Ritzman's recognized the need to provide education to satisfy the growing interest in natural medicines. Graf has also led the Ritzman's chain into a niche marketing venture — hormone replacement therapy (HRT). A survey of patients indicated that HRT and natural products were two areas in which to deliver pharmaceutical care. Graf later found that 90% of customers were happy with these new clinical services. Although the 90% gave Ritzman's pharmacists rave reviews, only 10 to 15% of them said they would pay for such services.

Today, Ritzman's continues its commitments by offering consumers seminars on many subjects. For example, a seminar on HRT is $10 per attendee and individual-counseling sessions with a pharmacist are $75 per half-hour session. Because of the dedication of Graf and his highly specialized support pharmacist, Ritzman's has many pay-as-you-go consumers attending seminars and individual counseling sessions.

Graf is much more than an employee. He loves being a pharmacist and finds joy in searching for ways to improve the business opportunities where he works. In describing his major influences Graf says:

Hard work is not an issue, I began working before I went into high school. While I may have missed some teen year events because of an after-school job, it set in place a work ethic where I learned a lot about the principles of managing a business, putting integrity into your work, the commitment it takes to build a business, and what it takes to market a niche product. Further, my dad was a CPA, we all heard a lot about business around the dinner table. His influence encouraged me to think about going to the University of Akron to get a business degree after high school. Then, when I was enrolled in my first year of college, Mr. Ritzman offered me a job in one of his pharmacies. After about a month I was promoted to his long-term care department where I put in forty-plus hours a week while remaining a full-time student. Then one day my dad remarked, 'Son, it looks like you really enjoy what being a pharmacist is all about.' I knew then I had found my professional home. After all, if Mr. Ritzman could talk five of his six sons into being pharmacists, there must be something in it. Finally, as I am someone who takes things very prayerfully, I knew Mr. Ritzmann had a door opened for me and I just needed to walk through it.

Graf transferred into pharmacy school at Ohio State University, and after graduation worked for 3 years in an independent pharmacy followed by another 3 years in a grocery chain pharmacy. But his desire to learn more about the business side of pharmacy remained. To satisfy that desire he returned to Ohio State where he enrolled in an M.S. program in pharmacy administration. It was during a special summer residency that he was assigned to Ritzman's Pharmacies. Upon graduation he returned to Ritzman's Pharmacies and has been there ever since.

When Graf talks about people who have influenced his professional decisions, he says, "The list is long, but it would include my dad, Ohio State pharmacy administration staff, a few professors from Ohio Northern, a junior high teacher, and a family friend, Tom Finley, who remains a friend and mentor."

Today, Graf is married with four children and likes to take them fishing when he has a day off from work. One tradition he has cultivated with his family is to take 2 weeks during Spring Break to a warm climate. Graf has recognized the need to relax and get away. "I never knew until recently how important it was to get those large blocks of time to recharge my batteries and to spend time with my children as a role model."

"To me," he says, "pharmaceutical care is a movement that has emerged as being the right chemistry existing between pharmacists and the public we serve. In fact, our mission statement says this in a special way." Today, under Graf's tutelage, Ritzman's Pharmacies offer a battery of specialized pharmaceutical care services including specialty compounding, home infusion, and disease management programs for cholesterol, diabetes, and asthma. Graf proudly states, "We have encouraged all our pharmacists and home nurses to help with program development and delivery. They each have areas of specialization. Our only obstacle to more growth in the pharmaceutical care arena is not finding payment sources among insurers, but that has not deterred us from our efforts to educate patients and convey our special knowledge to help them."

Also under Graf's guidance, Ritzman's publishes a bimonthly news-letter for all its patients and providers. These newsletters market Ritzman's natural product education seminars conducted at four of Ritzman's eight locations. Each seminar is open to the entire community and each lasts about an hour. These seminars cover subjects such as natural hormone replacement therapy, cooking with soy, Yoga, choles-terol management, diabetes management, and stress management.

Graf believes in being prepared for the day when pharmaceutical care compensation systems are in place. He requires all Ritzman's pharmacists to document the care interventions that they have given. As with all the patient programs he oversees, Graf has developed a short system to document all patient encounters and interventions. Copies of these charts are sent to the patient's physician. "Remember," says Graf, "the physician's pen is the source of all health care transac-tions, and because we are willing to document care we are now seeing physicians write prescriptions not only for medicines, but for us to counsel their patients about them as well. It has become very profes-sionally satisfying to get a prescription that reads 'patient has fibromy-algia and needs counseling from a Ritzman's pharmacist.' When we started sending copies of our patient counseling documentation to the patients' physicians in 1997," says Graf, "many physicians at first thought we were encroaching on the practice of medicine, so we invited the physician community to an open house in one of our facilities. They later thanked us, especially for carrying products that we believed in and also for not carrying products that had a less-than-stellar reputation or any hint of being ineffective. Today, local physicians know we care what our patients are taking especially over-the-counters or herbals and what medicines they have been prescribed and we have this documentation to back up the facts that we do care."

Graf earned an M.S. in pharmacy administration in the early 1990s. He continues to read avidly. "The types of books I read are closely related to business themes," says Graf. "I do not read books on the bestseller fiction list. What I find inspiring are autobiographies that give glimpses into peoples' achievements or lessons in life that they have learned. Recently I've been reading Robert Hargrave's *Masterful Coaching* and David Cotterrel on leadership." Graf goes on, "The more I read about how to work in today's business environment, the better I become at helping the Ritzman's team be successful."

> Remember, there is no more effort required to aim high in life, to demand abundance and prosperity than is required to accept misery and poverty.
>
> —Napoleon Hill

Graf does not hesitate to describe himself as a teacher, and as analytical and effective. "I don't dilly-dally around and I know people perceive me as being sincere and genuine," he says. "Further, I am also an honest guy and know that my basic honesty has been a critical element in my success. I get a good night's sleep when I am stressed, knowing that things will always look better in the morning."

Graf is also quick to state that although he enjoys the patient–pharmacist interface at the counter, he has learned that by grooming Ritzman's staff to help him meet their mission, many more patients can be reached. "I am not easily sidetracked and I know we have not been lucky in building a highly respected position in our communities. It has taken much discipline and hard work to reach a lot of people who believe in our committment to a community good."

Graf credits his wife for helping him realize more about his identity. He says that he never felt that his approaches to problems were unusual and knew that he was an intelligent person, but often his analytical side left people wondering if he was unapproachable. It was his wife who helped him work to overcome that impression.

ADVICE TO OTHERS

When asked to give advice to others who want to embark on the pharmaceutical care road, whether as a solo practitioner or an employee pharmacist, Graf has the following things to say:

- Focus on bringing out the good qualities in the people around you. After all, you are a member of a respected helping profession, and that means you should be helping patients as well as colleagues and other staff. When you help build your staff's success, your success will also fall into place.
- Focus on bringing a positive attitude into your work and life so you create an atmosphere where others can grow around you.
- Training and education are a smart investment in yourself and your colleagues. We are living in an era of empowered and enlightened consumers who are a force that can determine the outcome of a business because of their expectations.
- You can build a pharmaceutical care business by becoming the primary resource in the health care matters that are important to consumers. Satisfied consumers bring success to those from whom they have gotten help.
- Remember the words of Stephen Covey, as I found them true for me, "Your path will be personal and unique; everyone's is."

8

JUDITH SOMMERS HANSON: ENERGY AND FUN EQUAL PROGRESS

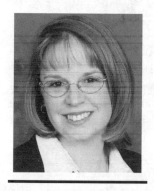

Judy Sommers Hanson

Ask Judy Sommers Hanson what her colleagues would say about her and there is no hesitation: "She has a lot of energy, is a lot of fun, very motivated, smart and hard-working. She does the job of two people even though she's paid for one." Talking with Judy you immediately agree. She is optimistic, enthusiastic, and full of life.

Do not take life too seriously. You will never get out of it alive.

—Elbert Hubbard

It has been a winning combination for her as she forges ahead building one of the strongest, most comprehensive and largest pharmaceutical care practices in the U.S. Dominick's in Buffalo Grove, IL, is a regional food store chain. Of its 140 stores, 92 have pharmacies. By 2001, about 5 years after she joined the company, 20 stores were working on providing pharmaceutical care services, 10 were actually seeing patients in formal programs, and 3 stores were offering comprehensive pharmacy services. Stores average 250 prescriptions per day and are staffed with two full-time pharmacists with 2-hour shift overlap and two pharmacy technicians per shift.

The company began exploring how to implement pharmaceutical care programs with Dr. Richard Hutchison at the University of Chicago College of Pharmacy in July 1996. They selected two busy locations that were part of their "fresh store" concept where pharmacies were located in the front of the store and had semiprivate consulting areas. Their philosophy was that if the pharmaceutical care model could work in busy stores, it could work in any store.

DEVELOPMENT THROUGH RESIDENCY PROGRAMS

Dominick's Pharmacies now have programs for asthma, diabetes, hypertension, hyperlipidemia, smoking cessation, osteoporosis, immunizations, and nutrition-wellness. Under the guidance of Judy Hanson and a number of community pharmacy residents, the programs have been developed and implemented incrementally. "Residency programs are a wonderful way to help patients, pharmacists, pharmacy students, and the company. Everyone wins," says Hanson.

Building up patient care services is a cornerstone of residency training. "Often residents can innovate outside the normal operational boundaries and infrastructure in a large company," she notes. "The residents are involved in whatever we are," Hanson says. "The best part is that two residents have stayed with us to continue building, refining and evaluating the pharmaceutical care practice." This is a clear example of a residency program's recruiting power.

"If you are interested in starting a residency, it is important to study what programs are out there and what your competitors are offering," Hanson asserts. "At Dominick's, we began the residency nearly 6 years ago. We studied the type of services being offered by our competitors and chose to focus our pharmaceutical care services accordingly." She thinks it is critical to understand your goals for starting a residency and to assess the internal environment as well. According to Hanson, one of the most important internal aspects of starting such a program is to gain upper- and middle-management support and involvement in the program's development. This helps to bring management expertise into the residency experience, which provides important guidance.

Grant support was received from both the APhA Foundation Incentive Grant program and the Institute for the Advancement of Community Pharmacy (IACP). Hanson encourages others to seek these opportunities to help support their ideas.

HOW SHE GOT THERE

Residency training was a key part of Hanson's own pathway to Dominick's. When she was graduated from the University of Chicago's College of Pharmacy in 1995, her career goal was to "take my clinical skills and expertise into the community pharmacy setting." She wanted to build on her education by completing an ambulatory care residency, but knew finding innovative programs would not be an easy task. Her search led her to the American Society of Health System Pharmacist (ASHP) Midyear Clinical Meeting. She was pleased to see a number of community pharmacy residencies listed in the residency matching program. After considering programs in Tennessee and Virginia, Hanson chose one sponsored by a Medicine Shoppe pharmacy owner in conjunction with the St. Louis College of Pharmacy. "I liked the fact that the residency was preceptor funded and the pharmacy owner was an assistant professor at the college. I also knew, as the first resident, I might not find the program overly structured and would have the opportunity to innovate."

And innovate she did. During the program, Hanson developed an asthma management service, refill reminder program, helped remodel the pharmacy, and researched computer systems to document care. While recruiting the program's next resident, she was approached by Dr. Hutchison. He explained the collaborative effort underway between the college and Dominick's and that the company was recruiting a pharmacist to serve as a residency preceptor and implement the pharmaceutical care program. She took the challenge.

NOT AN INNOVATOR?

In spite of her cutting-edge efforts, Hanson is humbled when people describe her as an innovator. "I think I am more of an overachiever," she reflects. Other words she feels describe her are teacher, professional, and motivator. She says she is still learning how to be a visionary. That said, she hopes the next 5 years will allow movement from a mixed position of dispensing and care toward one based solely on providing care services in a self-run private practice that is self-sufficient.

That sense of responsibility and leadership was learned growing up as the oldest child in a small family in the Chicago area. Helping her father in the printing trade taught her a strong work ethic that carried through in jobs at the local ice rink concession, selling shoes and clothing at retail stores, as a dormitory resident advisor and a pharmacy technician at Walgreen's.

The family is close-knit and Hanson's sister and brother-in-law are frequent traveling companions, joining Hanson and her husband, Dave, on adventures from San Francisco's Wine Country to Ireland's countryside. Dave's family is also in the area. They share similar family backgrounds and values, both of their parents are divorced and remarried. "I think they were content they had accomplished their mission raising their children," Hanson says. That shared experience shaped both Judy and Dave and contributes to the strong relationship they share.

BUILDING RELATIONSHIPS TO EDUCATE STAFF

Her ability to build good relationships has been a key to her success in implementing cutting-edge programs. "Educating the pharmacy staff on the vision — what we were trying to do and how it would change their work was the first thing we did. They were very receptive although a lot of reassurance was required," says Hanson. One helpful tip she offers in educating store managers about what the pharmacy is doing is to enroll them in the monitoring programs without charge. "We had two managers that were both hypertensive and they embraced the services, competing with one another on who had better control."

EDUCATING HERSELF AND TRAINING OTHERS

In addition to her college degree and residency, Hanson continued her education through APhA training programs in diabetes, asthma, and hyperlipidemia. She is working on obtaining her certified diabetes educator (CDE) certification as well. The college provides formal clinical skills and disease-related education for Dominick's pharmacists. Hanson educates the pharmacy technicians. "We provide pharmacists with a 13-module written program to develop clinical skills and learn lab values. We give them the materials up to 3 months in advance of a disease-specific program held at the college." During this component, pharmacists work in a patient care mode at the university's outpatient clinic for 1 or 2 weeks with mentoring from faculty. Pharmacists are told they are expected to go back to their practices and target a certain number of patients (usually 10) and physicians (usually 5 or 6) to get the services started.

Self-development is a higher duty than self-sacrifice.

—Elizabeth Cody Stanton

WORKFLOW CHANGES

Minimal workflow changes were made because most of the pharmacies have separate prescription inflow and outflow and semiprivate consulting areas. "We did learn that setting up appointments for initial patient assessment worked best during our 2-hour shift overlap." There were times when appointments needed to be made outside the normal shift, however, and being committed to getting things up and running was important to the task. Technicians do most of the phone triage, including refill permissions. They also have implemented an automated voice mail system to help manage workflow and dispensing priorities.

MARKETING TO PATIENTS

A number of approaches have been used to target patients, including telephone, letters, and in-store conversations. Refill reminder programs target patients on cardiovascular medications. Pharmacists call within a few days when patients fail to pick up their refill and also call a week ahead of time to remind a patient that a refill is due. Letters describing diabetes services were sent to patients identified from the dispensing database who were taking oral diabetic medications or insulin. "Corporate support was tremendous and was very helpful in allowing us to use the pharmacy dispensing database to target patients. We found working with patients in the store to be the most effective."

PHYSICIAN RESPONSE

Hanson reports, "The physicians do come into the pharmacy, and we find patients are very enthusiastic and speak with the physicians about the services they are receiving here." She adds that physician detailing is an important part of gaining their support for collaborative practice. Currently the team is focusing more on physician education and awareness building.

DOCUMENTING AND BILLING FOR CARE

To document care, the pharmacies initially used Carepoint's CogniCare software. "We found it too laborious, especially since it was not integrated with the dispensing system. Now, we document by hand, and I believe that really helps the pharmacist understand the pharmaceutical care process. We use templates with standard formats and flowcharts to put things in SOAP note format," Hanson says. They use a fee structure for services based on the RBRVS.

MISSION STATEMENTS

Judy Sommers Hanson guides her programs by adherence to well-thought-out mission statements (Figures 8.1, 8.2, and 8.3 below).

To provide patients with superior customer service when preparing and dispensing their medications. Our highly trained pharmacists in drug therapy management provide comprehensive patient counseling, education services, and medication monitoring to ensure safe and effective medication use. It is our commitment to help patients achieve better help through these services.

Figure 8.1   Mission Statement.

Our Diabetes Wellness Program is to provide patients with diabetes the knowledge, skills, and motivation needed to self-manage their disease on a daily basis to reach their desired target ranges of their glucose levels and minimize the complications from poorly controlled diabetes.

Figure 8.2   Mission for a Diabetes Wellness Program.

Through pharmacy-based cholesterol screenings, patient assessment, drug therapy evaluation, and patient education Dominick's Pharmacy Cholesterol Program will strive to: (1) identify patients at risk for heart disease and (2) assist patients in reaching and maintaining their target cholesterol levels.

Figure 8.3   Mission for a Cholesterol Lowering Program.

ROLE OF ORGANIZATIONS AND INFLUENCERS

Typical of Hanson's reliance on organizations to help drive progress, she thinks that the APhA has been very helpful. "They provide grant money, education, networking and most importantly, they have faith and support. I am especially glad to see they encourage students at all levels to be involved."

During her college days, Hanson was active in her sorority, Rho Pi Phi, and its community drug education activities. Now, she is an active participant at the National Community Pharmacy Association (NCPA), American Association of Diabetes Educators (AADE), the American Society of Consultant Pharmacists (ASCP), and APhA. Often you can see her on the educational programs of these groups, sharing the lessons she has learned in motivating others.

"Sharing is important. There have been so many people who have done so with me and it has made a huge difference," she reflects. Among them are the UIC externship coordinator, Avery Spunt, Professor Jan Engle, Debbie Harper Brown, and Barry Carter, now at the University of Iowa. "They talked about and demonstrated the aggressive role community pharmacists could play helping people. I knew from them that was what I wanted to do." Along with inspiring others as a team, she believes individual support on a professional and personal level is a key attribute in her success.

These experiences have led her to think constantly about "How can I get more pharmacists excited about doing this? How do I make it 'click' for them?" She hopes her colleagues and patients will remember her for her caring and willingness to take a risk. "I was one of the first people to do a community pharmacy residency. I wasn't afraid to take the risk."

We not only need to be willing to give, but also to be open to receiving from others.

—Anon.

ADVICE TO OTHERS

■ Love your profession and work hard. Be patient and enlighten the people around you. Persevere. You'll succeed one person at a time. Patients and other healthcare practitioners are interested — once they have the "Ah ha" experience, they become advocates.

- Be committed and don't be afraid to take on the challenge and the risk.
- When implementing pharmaceutical care, distinguish your role in providing care from your role in dispensing products. It will help others understand the difference and set you up well when you begin billing for services.
- If you are in a corporate setting, encourage nonpharmacy personnel and their families to avail themselves of your services. Many patients will go to store management and tell them how helpful and useful they find these programs.
- Network with others especially in pharmacy-related professional development programs. Colleagues are a constant source of motivation and support.
- Be involved. There are a tremendous number of programs and resources to support your transition.

People don't care about how much you know, until they know how much you care about them.

—Guy Flint

9

KELLEY HOFER: DESTINY IS A MATTER OF CHOICE, NOT CHANCE

Kelley Hofer is a positive person who believes that to go from happiness to fulfillment, we all have a choice of what side of the coin to look at — the one facing up or the one facing down. Hofer lives by this philosophy, which was first articulated by William Hubbard.

"There is something to enjoy no matter what you're doing in life," she says. "It really is up to you to decide how to view things." A perpetual optimist, Hofer bubbles with enthusiasm whether talking about her new child, her husband, her career, or her extended family. "One of the hardest things for me to see is depressed people. I just believe there is so much to be joyful about."

Joy is a common emotion around the Hofer household since the arrival of their daughter in late 2000. "She is so much fun and our lives have changed immeasurably for the better. When I stay up late thinking about something, it is usually 'What is my daughter going to be like when she grows up?' 'What will she do?' I just hope she will be as happy as her parents."

HUMBLE BEGINNINGS

Those same thoughts swirled through the heads of Hofer's parents while she was growing up in a small community of about 3000 in rural Washington State where her father ran a funeral home and her mother practiced nursing.

"It was a wonderful place for my brother, my sister and me to grow up," according to Hofer. "The community was very supportive of one another. People looked out for you and everyone had a chance to be involved. That kept a lot of us out of the trouble that many young people find themselves in today."

Hofer left to study pharmacy at the University of Washington and was graduated in 1993. Her mother's youngest sister was a pharmacist and a big influence on her career decision. "I knew I wanted to be a mom and pharmacy was appealing to me because of its flexible schedules, including less than full-time hours."

After finishing school, Hofer had no intention of working in the retail setting because she perceived there would be limited ability to use her clinical knowledge with patients. "I was burnt out on school and wanted to pay off student loans. Several women pharmacists I had met through the state association [Washington State Pharmacists Association (WSPA)] encouraged me to give independent pharmacy a try. So I got up the courage and began working with Elwin Blair at his pharmacy. It changed my life. I learned that I loved working with patients and that there was a lot of patient contact. I learned that there was a tremendous need to help people well beyond the dispensing function. If there was a defining moment in my career that led me to develop innovative patient services, this experience was it."

CREATING A CAREER

About a year and a half later she received an offer from the then 17-store Drug Emporium chain to be a pharmacy manager. "I enjoyed the business end of practice as well as the people end, so this seemed ideal for me as the next step toward creating my career." At Drug Emporium she began developing ideas for pharmaceutical care programs and found a receptive and supportive management team who were willing to let her innovate. She eventually developed a part-time pharmaceutical care coordinator position and her job was split between the new responsibilities and more traditional management ones. Drug Emporium started a hypertension management program and then services were expanded to include adult immunizations.

Hofer undertook immunization training in 1995 through the WSPA certificate program and began building services at one store. Eventually she had rolled out the program to include 50 trained pharmacists who were providing services at all 15 Washington stores. "We taught the other pharmacists through monthly manager meetings and by going directly to their stores. The majority of managers were very supportive and those that were not, were strongly encouraged to participate because this was the direction that pharmacy was headed."

She credits WSPA with much of her success. "Rod Schafer, WSPA's executive director, is such a positive and supportive person. He really helped keep me motivated during this time when challenges arose that might have truly set me back if I let them," she says.

She also credits her high school leadership class and its teacher. "That class was a major influence on me," she notes. "It provided an opportunity to do a lot of public speaking and gain confidence doing so. At Drug Emporium, we also were taught conflict management skills. These things combined I credit with giving me the skills I needed to sell myself and my ideas for new programs."

Creating and selling new and different programs that use her clinical knowledge and provide preventive care is what excites Hofer. She has built on her early success at Drug Emporium and now is using her experience at the Southwest Washington Medical Center, a 360-bed community hospital, where she has practiced for 3 years. Her road from community to hospital practice was influenced by another important life event — getting married. Her husband was transferred to Oregon with the forest products company for which he works, necessitating Hofer's departure from Drug Emporium."I knew how important a supportive management team was in being able to create and implement new services," Hofer says. "So, when I began interviewing for positions after we moved, I was very specific with what I wanted. Southwest Medical Center offered me the chance to continue to grow professionally."

CONTINUING NEW PROGRAMS AND CAREER DEVELOPMENT

At the Southwest Washington Medical Center Hofer manages smoking cessation services for employees of the hospital and is building an immunization component to their outpatient clinic offerings. Ultimately she would like to build a travel-vaccine clinic, where people who are going overseas and require a variety of vaccines against local illnesses can be immunized.

"Starting at the hospital, I was a little intimidated as it had been a while since I worked directly with physicians in a clinical setting. As a result, I decided to pursue my Pharm.D. degree through the university's external degree pathway. It has been one of the best things I have done." Now two thirds of the way through, Hofer says the 7 years of practice between receiving her first degree and enrolling in this program has made a huge and helpful difference.

LAUNCHING THE FIRST SERVICE

"The campus made the decision to become a smoke-free environment and wanted to offer smoking cessation help to those employees who wanted to take advantage of them. Smoke-free environments are a primary motivator for people to quit smoking. The enrollment in our employee smoking cessation program doubled as a result. We have achieved about a 65% success rate to date."

To effect the program, the human resources department provided nicotine replacement products for employees. The hospital was willing to reimburse the pharmacy for services because statistics show a $4000 savings for each person who stops smoking. Then, in March 2000 the program was expanded community wide. The community clinic charges $150 for the 6-week class and participants receive a $50 rebate if they succeed in quitting smoking. More recently, the local power company expressed interest in contracting with the community clinic to offer smoking cessation programs to its employees.

EXPANDING PROGRAMS

Within the inpatient immunization program, pharmacists identified there were a large number of older patients who contracted pneumonia. Hofer wrote a proposal to provide upon discharge pneumovax immunizations to patients over 65 years old. Most physicians were highly supportive of pharmacy's involvement. Hofer attributes that to the multidisciplinary approach of the project and the recognition that there are not enough physicians to provide all the preventive programs that are needed.

Pharmacists evaluate and educate patients regarding the vaccine, obtain their consent, and then order the vaccine. Letters are sent to patients' outpatient physicians for their clinic records. Vaccines are billed through the regular inpatient system.

Pharmacy residents and the ten inpatient pharmacists are trained to provide immunizations. Plans are to advertise the new service through the newspaper, health education flyers to the community, direct mail, and visiting people. Physician education and awareness is built through lunch meetings and direct mail.

REFLECTING ON SUCCESS

"I think getting along with people is probably the most important attribute for someone to succeed in this type of practice." In dealing with patients and physicians, Hofer believes that it is not possible to be successful if you don't know how or want to help others. Other key ingredients that make up the success mix are an ability to inspire others as a team, the ability to manage risk, and strong personal integrity. "You have to be able to build trust and that is fundamental to integrity." That is a key principle of Stephen Covey's — a book and training program she has read and appreciates.

Does she see herself as an innovator? Yes, in the sense that she is curious and likes to find things no one has done yet. She also sees herself as a teacher and a motivator. She likes to explain ideas to others and provide them with the skills and ability to carry through. She also describes herself as a professional and hopes that patients and colleagues would remember her as someone who truly cares about them and their health. When asked what her colleagues would say her strengths are, she replies, in typical humble fashion, "my outgoing nature and hilarious sense of humor, which I attribute to my mom." Her humility is apparent when asked about what she is proud of. "It is not myself that I actually am most proud of, but people who put care standards ahead of payment."

ADVICE TO OTHERS

What else besides being happy and having a sense of humor would Hofer recommend to others pursuing their pharmaceutical care dream?

- One thing leads to another. You just need to start with one thing and it will grow. Don't be intimidated by taking on too much too fast.
- Be involved and get educated.
- Avail yourself of the training programs and support networks that grow from them.
- Go the extra mile.
- Take on extra responsibility; you'll succeed and be rewarded.

- You will get shot down. You have to get up, brush yourself off, and do it again and again.
- A lot of people are waiting for the time to be perfect before they undertake programs, but there is never going to be a perfect time.
- You need to get out and play an active role in creating the opportunity.
- Find out what excites you. Do it and be thankful.

10

LAURIE KAUP: CARING FOR PEOPLE LIKE FAMILY

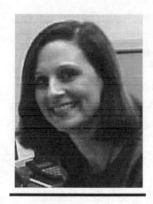

Laurie Kaup

Fort Recovery is a rural town of 1300 people located in western Ohio near the Indiana border. While Fort Recovery is 50 miles from any major town, it sits in a county of about 40,000 people known for their farms and agribusiness. It was here, 6 months after they graduated from Ohio Northern School of Pharmacy, that Jerry and Laurie Kaup decided they wanted to live. And, it was here that they began their special style of practicing pharmacy almost 20 years ago.

Their pharmacy is the only one in the downtown area of Fort Recovery. The location has two floors, including a 3000-sq. ft upper floor housing a traditional dispensary that fills 180 to 200 prescriptions per day and provides durable medical equipment (DME), and an equally large lower floor that is outfitted with a clean room and serves as the community's only source of home infusion services and custom compounding. The pharmacy is well known throughout the area. The staff of three hospitals and other medical specialists count on the Kaups to provide complete DME, home infusion services, asthma and diabetes monitoring, hormone replacement products, and hospice care services.

Laurie Kaup is especially proud is her diabetes disease management program. Since she initiated this program, more than 100 patients have enrolled. As part of this program, patients start with an initial appointment and with blood sugar and blood pressure tests. They then receive regular diabetic care flyers and are provided with telephone or in-store counseling every 6 weeks.

The Kaups have been successful in selling their pharmaceutical care services by hiring a full-time staff member with a marketing background. They also have nurses on staff. Documentation is done for services so patients can take a copy of the pharmacists "notes" to their physician. Charges for services vary, but they bill patients using an 80/20 rule. If the patient has insurance, he or she pays 20% out of pocket and the insurer gets a bill for the remaining 80%. Where appropriate, they use the HCFA 1500 forms for billing. "Since we are JCAHO accredited," Kaup says proudly, "we have a quality improvement committee that meets regularly comprised of patients and physicians who provide feedback on how we are doing."

To prepare herself and keep abreast of the latest developments in pharmacy, Kaup prides herself on the amount of continuing professional education she and her staff undertake. "I am particularly pleased that I undertook DME training with McKesson," she says, "because it was they who taught us how to bill for our time and work. In addition," she recalls, "I attend classes given by the Professional Compounding Centers of America at least two or three times a year. I also go to the American Medical Equipment Show once a year and the National Home Infusion Association meetings. Finally I make sure my 15 employees all attend at least one trade show per year."

How did Kaup get interested in being a patient-centered pharmacist? She cites her relationship with a cousin who had muscular dystrophy. "I always thought life was unfair to him," she states, "so I wanted to be helpful and involved in every aspect of patient care. Then when I was in pharmacy school, I took a job my first semester in a pharmacognosy lab. There I met a researcher who enlightened me on the politics of research and that convinced me I would be going into business. My dad was a CPA and he taught me a lot about business, but I owe my drive to my mother who always taught me not to settle for less."

In pharmacy school she met two men who changed her life. One was her husband and the other was her pharmacy administration professor. "My husband has a gift that has never failed — his ability to help me see the brighter side of life. My pharmacy administration professor gave me two gifts: a job right after graduation in his own pharmacy where I could learn the ropes, and 6 months after graduation, he helped arrange for our first inventory so we could open the pharmacy my husband and I run today."

To open their pharmacy, the Kaups borrowed $45,000 from a local businessman. "He was a local insurance agent, but he had faith in us and taught us what servicing the customer was all about as well as what life in a small town would be like." Kaup adds, "If we had not been able to make a business plan with 5-year projections per the instructions of our pharmacy administration professor, I am sure we would not have gotten the loan."

How does this busy pharmacist keep a balanced life? "When I have a day off I like to be with my kids. I usually take them to a sporting event. I like to golf and I like nature, particularly trees. It is my hope to write a book about the personalities in trees. I can see the personality of many of my friends and relatives when I contemplate a tree. Also, I love to have lunch with my mom or take a trip to visit my daughter."

Does Kaup ever take a vacation? "Oh, yes," she replies. "My husband and I believe in taking a big vacation with kids. As a result, our kids have been to China, Cancun, Australia, and such odd places as Slovenia. These are great family affairs that really allow us to reconnect."

Where does Kaup find the inner motivation to move forward? "I read a lot. In fact, I read every night before I go to bed. Recently, I read Don Blanchard and Don Schules, *The Little Book of Coaching*. I admire authors like Stephen Covey, Rick Bettino, and R.A. Burton (*Secrets of a CEO Coach*). My mom has introduced me to a speakers club which I like to attend and when I drive, I listen to National Public Radio." Kaup handles work-related stress by getting up at 5:30 a.m. and exercising in a nearby gymnasium with a neighbor.

> Persistence is the power that produces amazing achievement. Great efforts come out of industry and persistence; for audacity doth bind and mate the weaker sorts of mind.
>
> —Frances Bacon

Labels? Kaup believes the attributes she possesses that are most responsible for her success are her ability to work hard and persevere, her strong personal integrity, her mental toughness, and her vision. She relates, "I am always trying to create a vision of what I should be doing next. I am always trying to invent new ways to help people. I get energized from this and it is fun. Actually, I am afraid of stopping what I do because it is so much fun. For example, I can see how much help we are giving women because we started HRT [hormone replacement therapy] counseling and that is really fun. This would never have happened if I were not a pharmacist."

When a man is gloomy, everything seems to go wrong. When he is cheerful, everything seems right.

—Proverbs 15:15–17

What is next? Kaup says the fast changes in health care are a bit scary but she plans to persevere and motivate the staff to keep reaching.

ADVICE TO OTHERS

Laurie Kaup's advice to those who want to build a patient-centered pharmacy practice in the new millennium includes:

■ Make sure you have a rock-solid partner who can keep pushing you every day toward shared goals, and who is consistent in his or her behavior toward you, and who is comfortable enough in his or her relationship with you to give you the freedom to explore.

11

MAX PEOPLES: A CRUSADER WHO BELIEVES IN EDUCATED CONSUMERS

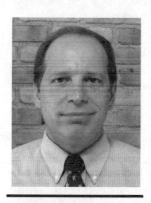

Max Peoples

"I had a grandmother who was a pharmacist. She learned pharmacy under the old apprenticeship system. She had a great heart and ran her own pharmacy for 30 years. When I was a junior in pharmacy school I read about the office practice pharmacy run by Eugene White in Virginia. These two influences convinced me I could survive in pharmacy, do it my way, and do as Grandma said, that is, to keep patients first."

Those who bring sunshine to the lives of others cannot keep it from themselves.

—James Matthew Barrie

Wanting to "keep patients first" and almost 3 years after his 1983 graduation, Max Peoples opened his 1100-sq. ft. Uptown Pharmacy in an upscale area of Columbus, Ohio. Prior to the opening he spent his first 2 years after graduation working for a community hospital and 8 months in a large independent pharmacy. He spent the time "learning the ropes" while he negotiated the purchase of the 100-year-old pharmacy that became his professional home. Today, Peoples has a staff of two full-time pharmacists, one part-time pharmacist, two pharmacy technicians, two clerks, two pharmacy students, and a resident Pharm.D. student. His pharmacy dispenses about 140 prescriptions and provides about three comprehensive pharmaceutical care consults per day.

In addition, the pharmacy offers immunizations, asthma, hyperlipidemia, and diabetes management services, an anticoagulation clinic, and specialty compounding. The pharmacy has two private counseling areas outfitted in mahogany paneling that are separated from the dispensing area. In the early years Peoples began doing diabetes management because it was one disease state that produces rapid changes in a patient's quality of life.

Uptown Pharmacy believes in having a shared mission. The statement is advertised in the local paper and on flyers to local doctors. In spite of that, Peoples believes, "Most customers arrive through the best advertising of all — word of mouth and referrals, as I get little physician support." What sets Peoples and his pharmacy apart is his belief that an empowered consumer is the best consumer. As such, his counseling includes not only advice on the drugs being prescribed, but on the therapeutic category involved, disease management risk factors, and anything that would help a patient take responsibility and an active role in his or her own care.

In addition to his grandmother Peoples believes the people who influenced him most are his parents and the values they instilled in him. "I also believe," he further states, "that I was influenced by learning about people who became heroes through personal sacrifice and perseverance. For instance, Susan B. Anthony, or Sally Hemmings, who persevered until she got her children their freedom, or any of the pioneers who created this country under great hardship."

Peoples says he is continuously re-energized by being a voracious reader. "I read everything in sight," he says. "From Tom Clancy to *National Geographic*, from a host of professional journals to the Sunday paper — I read a lot of human resource material because I know that is important to my success. I read all I can, as I never know where the next great idea may come from."

One great idea of which Peoples is proud is bringing a bar code scanning device, used to match a prescription product's national drug code (NDC) to the bottle of medication from which it is dispensed, to the marketplace. "Every pharmacist dreads the day he or she dispenses the wrong medication. Some research shows 2% of all prescriptions are subject to errors. I can show it is [really] as much as 7% … and that I have the tool to reduce or eliminate 75% of the mismatches between NDC numbers on the dispensing bottle and the prescription's product. It is very satisfying to me to know that I can help pharmacists ascertain they have the ointment in their hand when it should be the cream. These are errors to us, but are usually not realized as possibilities by the patient."

> The only certain measure of success is to render more and better service than is expected of you.
>
> —Og Mandino

When asked how he keeps from thinking negatively, Peoples replied, "I am not the kind of guy who lets things get him down. I find there is always a positive side to every event or a positive way to make something happen. If I cannot see a positive route to reach a goal, I am able to move on and not dwell on any negativity. Perhaps I was fortunate as a child to have a lot of reinforcement from my family and I had a lot of little successes, thus for me failure is not an option." He continued, "From the beginning of my professional journey into pharmacy I always knew that building a relationship with a patient was the only way to go. Thus, I never focused on myself. I knew I would never go broke if I held to the philosophy that I was in pharmacy because I wanted to be helping people. I knew that they would appreciate this more than if they thought they were doing me a favor by patronizing my pharmacy."

Peoples did not look to any particular professional society, publications, or guidelines to start or maintain his pharmacy. His philosophy is outlined in his mission statement and in the flyers he distributes to patrons and area physicians.

ADVICE TO OTHERS

Max Peoples' advice for those contemplating the professional practice life, either on their own or as an employee is:

■ Do not believe society is ready for each new pharmacist to start out as a mini-physician or old time apothecary. You yourself must determine the type of pharmacist you want to be. Equip yourself with the right education, tools, and attitude to bring to society.

- You should not let anyone stop you from being that pharmacist you envision yourself to be. If this means sacrifices, less money, or being a burr under someone's saddle, so be it.
- Pharmacists are true professionals. They should never have to compromise their ethics for the sake of a policy or job that does not match their professional judgment.
- If ever a pharmacist is stopped from spending that extra 5 or 10 minutes with a patient who really needs help, take it as a defining moment and walk away. Start your own pharmacy for the people who recognize the value you bring to their community.
- Anyone who has thought through what it takes to be their own boss will be successful. Making that happen entails first seeing yourself in the right place and then just plugging away until your education and training benefit each and every patient.

It takes 20 years to make an overnight success.

—Eddie Cantor

12

RICK MOHALL: MAKING A DIFFERENCE

Eckerd's Patient Care Centers are professional office-type pharmacy practices built at over 40 of their locations. The pharmacy in which Rick Mohall practices is more traditional, but has recently begun providing pharmaceutical care services in a diverse urban and densely populated Pittsburgh neighborhood.

Rick Mohall and Eckerd Drugs teamed up to provide a unique twist in pharmaceutical care services — two innovative demonstration projects that document the pharmacist's value in managing patients with asthma. While Mohall's involvement with these asthma programs is relatively recent, Eckerd Corporation has focused on developing patient care programs for a number of years through its Eckerd Patient Care Centers. Patient response has been overwhelmingly positive. The patient care center is a test site for the two projects: one with BC/BS and the other with the APhA Foundation. The BC/BS program has about 120 patients currently enrolled. The APhA Asthma Quality Improvement Pilot's (AQIP) goal is to have 30 patients per site.

HOW THE ECKERD PATIENT CARE CENTER CONCEPT EVOLVED

At Eckerd's patient care centers, rather than taking a disease-specific approach, Tina Lampe-Izaguirre, R.Ph., and her colleagues focus on comprehensive drug therapy management. "We realized that you need to focus on the whole patient because often there are multiple conditions at work and concentrating on one can at times create negative consequences in another," says Lampe-Izaguirre. "Syndrome X is a perfect example where a patient suffers from type II diabetes, hypertension, hyperlipidemia, and trunkal obesity. Insulin resistance is involved and treating only one aspect might exacerbate another."

Lampe-Izaguirre was recruited by the corporation several years ago to plan and implement programs at the Eckerd Patient Care Centers with another colleague, Karen Halvorsen. "It was a bit intimidating because we were starting with a blank piece of paper. We knew we were going to be located in the outpatient physician center, but that was about it. We designed the space, determined what services to offer, wrote brochures, and decided how to recruit patients."

They began with a series of brochures describing the comprehensive services as well as services with a disease-specific orientation. Building a patient base required time for Lampe-Izaguirre and Halvorsen to concentrate on teaching physicians in the center, as well as pharmacists at surrounding Eckerd stores near their Florida location. They also were able to target efforts by working with the corporate office to identify patients who might be good candidates for the new services. "We worked hard to build relationships with store managers and pharmacists and presented our services at the center as part of the team approach to helping patients. In addition to visiting every pharmacist at every store, we provided training to pharmacists at district meetings. Our efforts were well received. As a result, referrals began coming to the center from the stores."

PROVIDING, DOCUMENTING, AND CHARGING FOR SERVICES

At most centers services are provided on an appointment basis. Initial consults are scheduled for 40 to 60 minutes and include comprehensive medical history and drug therapy evaluation, including indications, efficacy, safety, and compliance. A drug therapy treatment plan is created and communicated to the patients and their physicians. Follow-up visits are generally 20 to 30 minutes. Point-of-care services to support drug therapy management are provided, including total lipids, coumadin levels, monofilament testing, and the like. Care is documented using the Assurance Patient-Centered Pharmaceutical Care Software from Health Outcomes Management, Inc.

In addition to the patient base built through detailing, Eckerd provides corporate support in generating contracts for services with HMOs and employer groups. Fees and billing for services are determined corporately with 80 to 85% of payments coming from third parties. The center transmits billing information using HCFA 1500 forms to Eckerd's corporate managed care group on a biweekly basis. Charges are based on the Medicare RBVRS — the same scale that physicians use.

At Mohall's pharmacy the service is being offered free-of-charge during the demonstration project stage, primarily because many surrounding hospitals provide free asthma education.

CREATING AND TAKING ADVANTAGE OF OPPORTUNITY

With Eckerd very focused on seeking new ways to demonstrate the value of the innovative services it was building, Mohall became involved when the company joined with BC/BS of Western Pennsylvania in June 1999 to test the impact of pharmaceutical care services on Medicare patients. Company management approached Rick because over his 22 years of service he had established a reputation as a "doer" with regard to patient care. He consistently sought ways to talk with seniors and others in his community about medication management, health care promotion, and other pharmacy topics. He was frequently involved in neighborhood health fairs and screenings as well.

"I have always enjoyed interacting with people and have found it fun to take the initiative to be involved in ways that I can communicate with patients," Mohall notes. Remember what leadership guru Warren Bennis says — that leaders are people who set out to live their lives fully, doing what they love to do. Rick Mohall is a great example of this principle. His initiative in finding ways to interact directly with people in his community led him to expand on that love to a much greater extent within a large company.

Your best shot at happiness and personal satisfaction is not earning as much as you can, but in performing as well as you can something you consider worthwhile.

—Anon.

BEING CREATIVE: STARTING THE BC/BS PROGRAM

"We have a traditional pharmacy and that was a challenge when we first began the BC/BS pilot," says Mohall. "We found whatever space we could to provide counseling, whether it was moving chairs into the pharmacy aisles or finding space in the back room somewhere. It didn't matter. We did whatever we had to do to make it work. I truly believe the key is for a patient to have a one-on-one relationship with the pharmacist."

Mohall's outgoing and collegial nature also helped him recruit patients for the pilot from his fellow pharmacists in surrounding stores. Like Tina, he reached out to explain what his pharmacy was doing and how it might lay the groundwork for further programs down the road. "Regardless of my personal relationship with my colleagues, it really made a difference in whether a patient chose to participate based on the relationship they had with the individual pharmacist," he says. Using the central database information to help target BC/BS patients, he would send the names of potential participants to the store they frequented, requesting that store pharmacist proactively reach out and recruit patients to the pilot. From the initial list of patients about 20% responded to contacts and 10% ultimately enrolled in the project.

Such numbers are typical of start-up programs. Mohall observed, as many others have, that success is built one patient at a time. Almost every text on pharmaceutical care agrees that this is true for nearly any new activity. The hardest part is to take the first step.

THE NEXT STEP: BECOMING AN APhA FOUNDATION ASTHMA QUALITY IMPROVEMENT PROGRAM (AQIP) SITE

Mohall says the AQIP program has been a great opportunity to work with pediatric asthma patients and build additional skills since much of the BC/BS work was with seniors. In this program, working with a child's parent or caregiver can be especially challenging — not only must you involve the child, but, depending on the child's age and abilities, clearly the caregiver also plays a large role in managing the child's condition. The goal is to recruit 30 pediatric patients, and, using his prior experience to assist with creative ways of getting patients to participate, Mohall was about halfway there when we spoke.

HARD WORK AND HELPING PEOPLE
ARE THE FOUNDATION

Both programs are examples of Mohall's 5-year vision for pharmacy. He hopes that one day these types of services will be usual rather than unusual in a pharmacy. This vision was shaped by his upbringing as an only child of Polish Catholic immigrants and forged by the values of hard work and helping people. "I was taught the importance of being dedicated to the work you chose and not to expect anything to be given without working for it," reflects Mohall. His parents are still living nearby and he helps them frequently as they age. "It has been difficult to see my parents decline and begin to suffer from disease. I often look at my patients, and frankly, I treat them the way I want my parents and kids to be treated." That approach has served him well in caring for both seniors and pediatric patients.

Mohall's first degree was not in pharmacy, but in biology from Pennsylvania State University. "I really like the area of western Pennsylvania where I was raised, and did not have the desire to travel far beyond it to school. I had always liked and done well at math and science so decided to study biology. I had hoped to combine that with a medical career because I am a people-oriented person. A friend suggested I look into pharmacy and that was it." He was accepted to all four Pennsylvania schools of pharmacy but chose Duquesne because of its religious nature and location. While there, he married his wife, Sandy, whom he had met in high school. They enjoy the company of their two children who are 12 and 18 years old.

INTERACTING WITH PEOPLE: A CRITICAL FACTOR
IN JOB CHOICE

After doing his rotations in various community and hospital practice sites, it became clear that an environment where interacting with patients was possible would be important in deciding where to work after graduation. "I worked at Beacon Pharmacy 30 hours per week during school. The pharmacy served nursing homes too. I was able to set up a unit dose system as an intern and was involved in developing and conducting nursing in-services. That experience tilted me toward community practice."

Shortly after, Thrift Drug opened a mail-order operation and asked for volunteers. At that company, a pharmacist serves as general manager, running both the pharmacy and the store. The concept appealed to him and so Mohall took advantage of the opportunity and parlayed it into community involvement. He talked frequently with senior groups and enjoyed being a source of information.

BUILDING SKILLS

But just wanting to be in an interactive environment did not automatically lead to success. Communication skills and patience are critical. So is patience since most programs take longer to develop than planned. Mohall's high school and college jobs, working long, demanding hours on a road crew and telemarketing magazines, were great skill builders in this regard. "In telemarketing, if you completed 5 of 80 calls a night, that was a success and the boss was thrilled," he recalls. "In most work, that would be a failure! I learned communication skills and caught on quickly that you need to choose your words and how you say them very carefully."

PLAYING HARD IS IMPORTANT TOO

In addition to working hard at the pharmacy and with the innovative demonstration projects, Mohall plays hard, too. "My father always kept his sense of humor and perspective and taught me that too. He's very upbeat about living. In my house, we like to do many, many things as a family from taking in a movie or a play, to going to sports events, or playing sports ourselves. Season tickets to the Pittsburgh Pirates are a highlight of the summer; so are occasional weekend ventures to the beach or concerts." Family vacations figure prominently; Disney World and Myrtle Beach are favorite spots. "I'm a pretty simple person," he says in typical humble fashion. "I can do just about anything to unwind from the pharmacy from reading the newspaper to catching a game on TV."

That simplicity and sincerity is evident when asked how he wants his patients and colleagues to remember him. "I just want them to know that I cared about making their lives better." He is grateful that they came to trust his opinions and suggestions about their therapy.

ADVICE TO OTHERS

- The key is wanting to help people. Be involved with patients and they'll respond. "I have had patients say, 'You saved my life,' or 'You are an angel of mercy.' They are incredibly grateful."

- Be a good listener. Hear and address the patient's concerns. Then fix them. It is not easy, but over time you acquire the skill.
- Be patient and persistent. You will see people you want to help, but for any number of reasons are unable to as much as you'd like. Don't get discouraged.
- You need to spend money to make money. You need to decide to pursue this type of practice and stay with it.
- You cannot pursue patient-oriented practice for the paycheck. If you are a clock-watcher, this type of practice won't work for you.
- Start by asking, "Is this how I can make a difference in my chosen profession?"

13

BEVERLY SCHAEFER: A FEMINIST CHILD OF THE 1960s BECOMES A LEADER

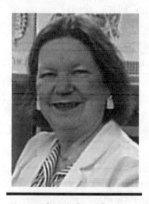

Beverly Schaefer

In her typical straightforward, shoot-from-the-hip manner, Beverly Schaefer says about her decision to be a pharmacist, "It paid well. I wanted to do something in the medical field. I learned I enjoyed people [while] working in the neighborhood theater during high school. But nurses' salaries were poor. Medical school cost too much. I wanted a job where I could support myself without relying on a man; to be able to depend on myself in the event I was abandoned." That strong sense of self was imparted growing up in a blue-collar family. The oldest of three girls, Schaefer and her sisters were raised to feel empowered and were taught that girls could do anything that boys could.

She attended the University of Washington's pharmacy school, graduating in 1970 in a class that was 33% women, among the highest in the country. "Washington has always been a very progressive state," she notes. It was the ripe environment for change and the mentoring of Don Katterman, a professional who was passionate about and involved in pharmacy, that led her to pursue a career in community pharmacy practice. "He believed pharmacists should get paid for services. I'm not sure if that grew from his observations during his 4 years as a Squibb sales representative or elsewhere," she says. He gave her a real heads-up on what was happening in the profession, exposed her to new ideas, and told her that many would disagree with the new way of thinking. Another key influence at that time was the school's assistant dean, Louis Fisher. "He was a much-beloved, roly-poly, jolly man who really tuned into the student's thinking," she reflects.

JOINING A PRACTICE

It seemed natural to join Katterman in his pharmacy after graduation. The 3800-sq. ft. pharmacy was in a stable, family, urban neighborhood on the edge of two affluent areas in northeast Seattle. In addition to herself and Katterman, there was a "drug clerk," as they were then known, Juanita, who came to them with 30 years of chain pharmacy experience and savvy. They spent their time "retailing, selling, and providing care."

In 1975, they expanded the store, and again in 1985, to its present 5600 sq. ft. Its space is split about evenly between the pharmacy and front end. It is unique thanks to the contribution of a designer hired to help lay it out. The pharmacy was set diagonally, however, rather than the typical straight-across-the-back-of-the-store design. There is a large gift area in the front with a big gazebo. This houses top-of-the-line and high-end gift items, including perfumes, crystal, stuffed animals, and the like. "It definitely has ambience," she says. "We did make a mistake with a raised pharmacy, which we eventually changed."

The pharmacy is open from 9 a.m. to 8 p.m., Monday to Friday, 10 a.m. to 6 p.m. on Saturday, and 12 to 5 p.m. on Sundays. There are two full-time pharmacists, three part-time pharmacy students, and a pharmacy assistant. "We haven't gone the pharmacy technician route because we have always had students. People really like that."

She continued the tradition after Katterman's death in 1982 at age 54. His wife kept the store open with Schaefer and Juanita running it. At the same time, Schaefer had just given birth to her second child, and a former student, Steve Cone, worked relief for her at the pharmacy. The few months she took off to be with her growing family was the only time off she has ever had. When she returned from her leave, Steve Cone stayed on. They purchased the pharmacy in 1996. "The response to Don's death was amazing. We had three customers offer to buy the store so we could continue to run it. Many pharmacists offered to help us. Don's wife realized the pharmacy community was her home too, as it had been Don's. She was involved in the National Community Pharmacists Association (NCPA) auxiliary that year too. [Don's wife] wasn't ready to give that up. [The store] was financially sound enough to keep the pharmacy open. We ran it like we always ran it," she notes.

"I remember there were challenges, however," Schaefer continues. "We ran out of narcotic blanks which, of course, we discovered the same week we switched wholesalers. Then we ran out of labels. It was a real experience, learning as we went."

Just remember when you think all is lost, the future remains.

—Robert H. Gadded

For the things we have to learn before we can do them, we learn by doing them.

—Aristotle

IT IS ALL ABOUT FAMILY

But, they survived and flourished. Schaefer and her husband, Michael, raised their daughter Katy, who was born in 1977, and son John, who was born in 1982. She and Michael met while in college. Schaefer says that Michael, a forest and park planning major, has been a very atypical breadwinner with stints volunteering and as a part-time zookeeper. He and John spent a lot of time doing wilderness drawings and building projects. It is reflected in John's mechanical nature and talent at building model cars.

Katy, on the other hand, eventually majored in business, having been undecided until her junior year of college. "She's really good with people and has a flair for retailing, marketing, and accounting," Schaefer adds proudly. "It was great to have her work at the store." She reflects that having children was the best decision she ever made. At the same time, it is the hardest, most demanding, most expanding job in the world. "It is nice to still like them as adults after growing up as a family. We didn't have hard teenage years."

THE BUSINESS CHANGES

"I remember in January 1994 when we signed a major third-party contract moving from usual and customary to a card program with a significant AWP discount. Steve and I really began to wonder what it meant for the business. How much further could and would reimbursements go? We began to really analyze the business and ask ourselves would we rather be dispensing 200 prescriptions a day at $2 profit each or 100 a day at $5? We decided on the latter. We sent 300 families out the door who had that plan — in a neighborhood pharmacy! These were powerful, influential families. We knew we needed a powerful reason."

It took a lot of courage, but they explained that insurers were not paying enough, that they had a different philosophy than the major prescription insurers, and that as patients they were not getting what their doctors wanted them to have. They positioned the pharmacy as a partner to the patients, explaining that if they changed insurance, they would consider filling the prescriptions again. Most families took their prescription business elsewhere, but still came to the store. "We told them to go where they had to go to get their commodity, but when they needed health care, to come here," she recalls.

The greater the obstacle, the more glory in overcoming it.

—Molière

This led Schaefer and Cone to create a new vision of practice over a 6-month transition period to a different product and service mix. Part of that was spurred on by a particularly nasty protracted lease negotiation. This led them to search for new revenue streams. In January 1995 she went to a Washington State Pharmacist Association (WSPA) Midyear Meeting where she attended a session conducted by a panel of pharmacists on immunizing in pharmacies. "I thought, if they can do it. I can do it." Thus, they began on the path toward patient-care services.

"I have the best partner in the whole world. We have very complementary skills. He lets me go out and observe and learn. I'm the entrepreneur, networking, going to talks and such. Steve is the back-end support, running the finances, the rock. He is very supportive of the new ideas I bring back and [which] we try to implement."

THE TRANSFORMATION STARTS

Schaefer and Cone physically reconfigured the pharmacy and removed durable medical equipment (DME) from a 20 × 20-ft space. They brought in two 5 × 5-ft walls, two chairs, and a table. Schaefer hung their training certificates and started giving flu shots there in the fall.

Customers watched and talked about the remodel during the summer. It provided Schaefer and Cone the chance to educate their customers on what was happening. They tried to get them to look at things in the pharmacy in a different way and get them mentally ready for something new.

The most difficult part of the project was getting the collaborative practice agreement in place with a physician. She found they had to do a lot of homework, including which physician to approach. "We had many physician customers and friends, but we wanted to do it right. We wanted to figure out who would be the most antagonistic and what his or her concerns would be." They learned those fears centered on taking patients away, liability, training, and protocols.

They made an appointment and met with a neighborhood physician who was very involved in the community. After not hearing from him, they called again 10 days later. They learned of and addressed his concerns and eventually moved ahead. "It was a good learning lesson for us. For any new project, we take small, incremental steps."

All told, it cost about $1500 to get the program ready — about one third each for furniture, training, and supplies. They needed 300 patients to break even. After the fourth day, they made a sign for the pharmacy's front window: Flu Shots Here. People poured through the door. They treated the immunizations like new prescriptions, adding them into the regular workload. It forced Schaefer to get out from behind the counter. "There were so many surprises along the way. I reeled from the experience and it was all good," she remembers. By the end of the flu season, they had given 1000 shots.

Schaefer says, "Sitting down with customers and patients in that newly created space was enlightening. I learned so many things from them that really advanced the course of what we were doing. For example, I learned people loved the convenience of the neighborhood pharmacy and getting care evenings and weekends. That they could drop in without appointments. They began asking me what else we did. I asked them, "What else do you want us to do?" She realized there was a huge body of health care desired and needed, but not being provided by anyone. "It was when I finally lost my victim mentality about ratcheting reimbursements and how bad pharmacy was, etc."

It is better to know some of the questions than all of the answers.

—James Thurber

Optimism is an intellectual choice.

—Diana Schneider

THE NEXT STEPS

From those humble beginnings the practice has grown into one that offers cholesterol/lipid, HgA1C, osteoporosis, and PSA (for prostate cancer) screenings and emergency contraception services. They are appealing to fellow baby boomers who are "fat and forty," helping them make better and long-term lifestyle choices. It still "looks like and feels like you are gathering around someone's dining room table," she says. "People want personal attention." Their mission is to help people make wise decisions to maintain or improve their health.

Not he who has learned much is rich; but he who gives much.

—Erich Fromm

The osteoporosis service not only provides screenings at Katterman, but also at other pharmacies. When they researched the equipment needed, they decided to purchase instead of lease. They were able to break even on the $20,000 investment in 2 years by teaching other pharmacists to use it at their own stores, creating a portable machine and activity. "Here, in particular, is a huge population who may think they're well that no one is dealing with. They will pay for the services." Charges started at $25 per test. When deciding what to charge, she recommends pharmacists put things in perspective of other personal care services. For example, if they think $35 is too high, you can remind them that this is less than most people pay for a haircut.

They document care through a creative and self-developed at-a-glance text/graphic tool. It is easy to interpret and meaningful. The results are sent to patients' physicians with a cover letter. "We learned early on, if you take a public health approach to the services you are providing, physicians have a hard time arguing against them." They find the vast majority of patients come to the pharmacy for services before they go to their physician. All at-risk patients identified through the various screenings are referred to their physicians for treatment.

ATTRIBUTES OF SUCCESS

Schaefer believes her enthusiasm is key to her success, along with the ability to spot trends and network with vendors and customers. When she's not working, she enjoys winding down with a good book — biographies, business, and fiction. She also takes her enthusiasm on the road and tries to plan a spontaneous adventure for a few days before or after the association meetings in which she participates. At last count she has visited 45 states.

Happiness is found along the way — not at the end of the road.

—Anon.

Her goal is to move others by sharing her insights. She has a unique point of view into the relentless demands many typical community pharmacists face, which keep them from making any new plans. A good network of peers can help. While organizations and schools try to help, she still finds it best to learn from those who have accomplished a task and can tell you how to get from point A to B to C in a practical manner. Yet she feels it is naive to think that all practitioners will want to change and become caregivers.

"I don't have aspirations to climb anywhere or have a big house. I hope people remember me for being trustworthy and wise. We pride ourselves on the fact we serve our neighborhood. We want to continue to serve the neighborhood but in new and different ways, evolving our services to meet their needs."

ADVICE TO OTHERS

- Decide you are going to move into patient-care services and make it your priority.
- Say yes. This is real life. You just do it. When you don't have a choice, you do it.
- Be an independent thinker. Try to decide what your goal is for the service you want to offer.
- Start simple. Take it one step at a time. Work on it a little bit each day.
- Nothing is forever. If you make a wrong choice, you can always change your mind.
- Change with it, in spite of it, keep going on.
- Step out from behind the counter. It is amazing what you'll see. I loved it. So did the patients.

14

DIANE SCHULTZ: INITIATING INNOVATIVE SERVICES

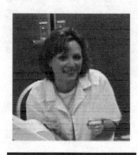

Diane Schultz

Who would have thought that sorority rush would be a defining moment for Diane Schultz? But it was during that process at Washington State University in Pullman that they kept asking her, "What is your name and major?" That is when Schultz was introduced to the idea of becoming a pharmacist. "I liked math and science and I had thought about becoming an engineer, but people interaction was too important. I was focused on health care but did not want to work in a hospital because the environment felt too confining and I felt I could make more of a difference out working in the community." She talked with a career counselor and to WSU pharmacy professor Keith Campbell and her mind was made up. Schultz has forged ahead implementing numerous services in the independent and chain pharmacy environment.

TRYING NEW THINGS

"I really like having the ability to innovate and try new things," says Schultz. "I am … fortunate that I've worked with supportive pharmacy directors who have allowed me to do so." In her current position as pharmaceutical care coordinator with Long's Drug Stores, she is continuing to pilot asthma and diabetes pharmaceutical care programs.

She is also starting a travel immunization program. Prior to Long's purchase, the stores were part of the Drug Emporium franchise and had implemented hypertension, immunization, and emergency contraception programs. In fact, it was Schultz who hired Kelley Hofer (see Chapter 9) to develop these programs.

"When I started with Drug Emporium in 1991 as a manager, I was able to work with two other stores.... When Doug Callihan was brought in as the new pharmacy director from Fry's Food and Drug of Arizona, he asked me to become a supervisor. I hesitated. While I knew operations, I was afraid I would miss patient contact."

That is when Schultz talked with Callihan about implementing an immunization program, following up on a Washington State Pharmacist Association's (WSPA) educational training program she had taken. He responded enthusiastically. So Schultz brought in Hofer and trained two other pharmacists. In 1996 they gave 200 flu shots. By 1997, 15 other pharmacists were trained. "Customers were delighted. No one asked why pharmacists were administering immunizations, they trusted us," she reflects.

GETTING THERE

Building on her love of people is what led Schultz to the opportunity to innovate. She attributes her ability to get along with people and her love of the profession as key attributes of her success. After graduating with her B.S. in pharmacy in 1986, she cut her teeth working for a few years with the Sav-On/Osco chain after moving to Los Angeles. It was an interesting time, as the chain was converting to computers and the pharmacists she worked with were three elderly gentlemen who had never touched one before. It gave Schultz the chance to provide support and hand-holding to them through the change, reflecting her skills as a teacher — one of the labels she applies to herself, along with innovator, motivator, and professional.

LIFE-CHANGING EVENTS

In 1989, Schultz moved to Seattle. She wanted to expand her horizons beyond her solid chain pharmacy experience so began practicing in an independent pharmacy. The owner of the store was not a pharmacist, but he was very supportive of trying new things. During the year and a half that she was there, she lectured at the retirement home across the street and visited physician offices to help drum up business. But the business was reaching the end of its life, and about the time she decided to leave the owner sold. That is when the opportunity arose at the small franchise that was part of the Drug Emporium chain, allowing the chance to individualize store services in the marketplace. "Drug Emporium was known for filling a lot of prescriptions, but their culture was what attracted me. It had autonomy stamped all over it which was very exciting to me."

Her side trip to independent pharmacy proved to be a life-changing event for Schultz, but not in the professional sense. An ophthalmologist with whom she had developed an excellent working relationship recommended the store to his son who had been prescribed some medication. He came to the pharmacy and Schultz became his pharmacist. It wasn't long after on Valentine's Day when he sent a dozen roses — half in appreciation as a patient and half in appreciation as a friend. They began dating and eventually married.

CHARTING NEW TERRITORY

Schultz was charting new territory as a wife and in her new position at Drug Emporium. With the initial immunization program becoming a great success, Drug Emporium management allowed her to move ahead, implementing emergency contraception services in 1997. She worked with physicians to create collaborative practice arrangements with prescriptive authority. She was able to secure a grant to fund program marketing, and in the first year alone they saw 3500 patients in the 18 stores (of 24) where services were offered. They charge patients $35 for the service and treat it like a prescription, moving it efficiently from a workflow standpoint. It takes about 10 minutes to counsel the patients. Payment comes from cash, Medicaid, and pharmacies using HCFA 1500 forms.

OTHER SERVICES

Hypertension was the first service implemented. They chose it because taking blood pressures was not complicated. A pamphlet was created and used to market the service to patients and physicians. They faxed the brochure to physicians and followed up by phone. A $20 per month fee was charged for four weekly appointments and unlimited blood pressure readings. While there was a lot of interest, many people did not see the value in paying for the service and it was difficult getting it off the ground. So they installed blood pressure monitoring machines in each store and discontinued the fee-paying service.

They also have a cholesterol screening service that started 3 years ago at all the pharmacies. They have a cholestech machine that is shared among stores and each store offers screenings two times per year. Fifteen pharmacists have been trained to provide the services and charges vary from $10 to $35 per screen depending on the panel. HCFA 1500 forms are submitted and patients also receive receipts in the event they would like to submit them for insurance reimbursement directly.

LONG'S

In July 1998, Long's Drug Stores of California purchased the Drug Emporium chain. Schultz stayed on in operations, assured of the company's commitment to maintain patient-care programs based on Drug Emporium's initial success. In spite of that, it took about 2 years for her to realize that with all of the daily operational issues to attend to, patient-care programs always got put on the back burner. Schultz decided to leave the company to pursue what she enjoyed most. Long's asked her to stay. Her requirement was that management of the company had to be committed to pursuing pharmaceutical care service programs. Long's was and Schultz assumed the district responsibility for these initiatives. She feared losing touch with pharmacists in the field, so she created a position where she could spend 10 hours per week dispensing prescriptions and talking with the pharmacists.

"Long's has a good workflow system and many excited pharmacists," she notes. "Building relationships with pharmacists at the store level was critical to successful new programs. They are my friends and we respect one another. Our job is to work hand in hand to help people."

DIABETES/ASTHMA PILOT PROGRAMS

New programs are being developed in the diabetes and asthma arenas. Diabetes is unique in that it combines both a significant product and service component. It is a program that helps to meet the store or regional manager's bottom-line goals, which have been obstacles to developing pharmaceutical care programs. Why diabetes? Flash back to Keith Campbell, Schultz's WSU professor, a person she admires. She says, "He is diabetic yet is so positive about managing it." He represented both patient and professor to her. "He was funny, supportive and like a father to me — a real inspiration."

During her years of practice she also had a profound experience. She went to talk to a diabetes support group and from that activity, three patients began to come to her store and use her as their primary pharmacist. Shortly after, she transferred to a different store 15 miles away and all three of those patients followed her. "It showed me that I could make a huge difference in people's lives," she says. It was a defining moment in her development as a pharmacist.

The diabetes pilot was scheduled for launch in two stores with five patients waiting to enroll. Operationally excellent locations were selected, where pharmacists had good attitudes and interest in being role models by providing services. "Many pharmacists need and want training, and that is the first step," she notes. She has taken advantage of WSPA, manufacturer, and NIPCO training programs.

The diabetes program will be structured with an appointment system. Appointments will be offered 2 or 3 days per week during pharmacist shift overlap from 2 to 4 p.m. They will be documented using SOAP note format, and eventually billed using HCFA 1500 forms. They also offer group sessions and have developed a community talk to deliver to diabetic support groups.

The asthma pilot services are being implemented in one store in a low-income neighborhood. Garnering her colleagues' respect and further support, Schultz will often work dispensing prescriptions while the pharmacist provides care services. It is a good example of another attribute she feels has contributed greatly to her success — the ability to inspire others as a team.

Payment continues to be an obstacle and the programs have not implemented billing software at this time, relying on hand billing for now. With the asthma service, however, BC/BS will soon pay for services.

WORKFLOW CHANGES AND PROCESSES

There are separate drop-off and pick-up windows at the pharmacy counter. The use of color-coded clips helps with high-status items. They use a 3:1 technician-to-pharmacist ratio. Every store has a stand-up counseling station while six others have a sit-down counseling area.

TAKING THE HIGH ROAD

"I never saw myself as a leader in pharmaceutical care," Schultz says. "I didn't think I would be first among pharmacists. I just like to watch things come to fruition." It is typical of her humble and sincere nature. She is an empathetic individual and believes that is her greatest strength. "I think I developed it with my grandparents. I always was attracted to working with elderly people and, as their pharmacist, I was often the only person they would talk to during the day." She enjoys spending time with her 93-year-old grandmother and 98-year-old great aunt.

She appreciates the role even more now that she is the mother of two young children. Being a parent is what she's most proud of and wanting to see her children succeed is what often occupies her mind. "Family is what I care about most. Having a balance in life between work and family is critical to me." A few years ago, she found both herself and her husband focused on business. They had a full-time nanny and were no longer using their boat, even though boating had been a favorite hobby. "I realized one of us had to stop. I knew my job, felt I had achieved many successes, and was proud of what I'd done. So I decided I could step back." She has never regretted it.

> How different our lives are when we really know what is deeply important to us, and keeping that picture in mind, manage each day to be and to do what really matters most.
>
> —Stephen Covey

Schultz handles a busy life by taking care of herself with a regular exercise routine, visiting extended family, traveling to California and Arizona to keep up with friends she met while living there, and reading and learning. "I'm like a sponge. I try to soak up everything I can on how to be the best person I can be." Two books she has read and recommends to others along that line are *Transitions* by William Bridges and *Circle of Sympathy* by Celia Andrews.

Her driving force is to help people become self-sufficient and motivated. "When I design a program, I bear in mind that it has to be simple to implement at store level." The information she provides to pharmacists allows them to move their practice forward, focusing more on patient care. "Not all pharmacists accept this challenge, but it is very powerful when people trust you. In the end they feel more satisfied professionally and personally, because they see the difference they can make." She has been able to help many by implementing her life philosophy to balance what is important and sharing that with others.

There is no comparison between that which is lost by not succeeding and that which is lost by not trying.

—Francis Bacon

ADVICE TO OTHERS

- If you don't feel supported in your goal to focus more on patient care in your practice setting, ask yourself, "What could I do tomorrow when I walk in the pharmacy that I don't need permission for?" Schultz once made such a list with 40 items on it.
- Networking is a huge, positive support. It allows you to learn from others without recreating the wheel. State and national associations are a good place to start.
- Be persistent. If one person/patient says no, try another avenue.
- Keep it simple, especially when you are just starting.
- Find balance in your life among the things most important to you.

15

MICHELLE SHIBLEY: DOING MORE

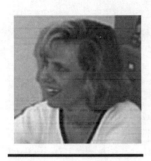

Michelle Shibley

When Dan Herbert, F.A.C.A., opened Richmond Apothecaries little did he know that his style of practice would eventually result in a partnership with his two daughters, Michelle Shibley, Pharm.D., and Catherine Cary, Pharm.D. Today they manage the Richmond Apothecaries group of pharmacies — Bremo-Westhampton, Metropolitan, and Henrico — located in the Richmond, VA area. The staff includes four full-time and one part-time pharmacist. Two clinical pharmacists, Shibley and her sister, provide pharmaceutical care services at all three pharmacies. Richmond Apothecaries also hosts a half-time pharmacy resident who provides additional clinical services. The three Richmond Apothecaries vary in size — 500 sq. ft., 1100 sq. ft., and 3000 sq. ft. They serve a diverse population ranging from indigent Medicaid patients to affluent professionals. Each pharmacy has semiprivate or private counseling areas and carries little front-end merchandise. Each pharmacy is known for its pharmaceutical care services that are integrated within the dispensing process. Current programs are in diabetes, asthma, hypertension, and comprehensive medication review.

According to owner Dan Herbert, it was his children becoming pharmacists that inspired him to expand the business and innovate. "When Michelle and Catherine decided to become pharmacists, then graduated in 1992 and 1995, I knew I wanted to ensure the practice would be there for them in a form that allowed them to practice at a high professional level." Herbert gathered his pharmacists for a weekend retreat where they brainstormed about what direction the pharmacies should take. "That started us on the right path," he notes. "It was like magic with constant ideas, changes, and energies put into developing clinical programs. Things really began to percolate and gather steam in the mid-1990s, and today we are comfortable developing clinical concepts and implementing them."

"I am so fortunate to have the freedom and flexibility to try things," says Shibley. "We've started some programs and discontinued others — things are constantly changing, but our commitment to the goal of providing quality patient care remains the same." In fact, Richmond Apothecaries was among the first pharmaceutical care innovators and served as one of 16 experts in the APhA and NWDA Concept Pharmacy research and education program. This program is dedicated to fostering pharmaceutical care innovation among pharmacists and understanding among policymakers, consumers, and other stakeholders.

A unique aspect of Richmond Apothecaries' approach to service is its strong integration with the dispensing process. "The dispensing process is critical in building a pharmaceutical care patient base and allowing pharmacists to identify program patients during each visit," says Herbert. A method was created to code patient records in the dispensing system so the pharmacist filling the prescription could identify the patient as part of a care program. Concise, disease-specific evaluation tools were created for the pharmacist to use during these visits. The pharmacy's clinical staff then reviews the information from the evaluation and comprehensive follow-up visits are scheduled. Patient visits consist of the pharmacist asking patients a list of prepared questions. Often this results in a letter being sent to their physician.

Richmond Apothecaries' pharmacists document their findings in a system using the SOAP format. They own a pharmaceutical care software program but have not found it as useful as a Microsoft Access database applied to meet their specialized in-house documentation needs.

Shibley views collaboration with physicians as a key component for their long-term success. "It is a cornerstone within each area of services that we have developed. For example, with our asthma program, we are lucky to be located next to a specialist with whom we have an excellent relationship. Referrals are frequent. We developed a number of these relationships when we implemented our hypertension program, but in the beginning referrals lagged." They found that while physicians did view their services favorably, making referrals to a pharmacy was outside their normal routine and they simply forgot to pursue it. The pharmacists persisted, resulting in more referrals and program growth. "We stay in touch with physicians by faxing a follow-up note from the pharmacist on each patient as we see them,"Shibley reports.

The Richmond Apothecaries Diabetes Care Program was developed using a collaborative approach and as part of an APhA outcomes-based research project. The 12-month project measured self-monitored blood glucose results, adherence with medication among a group of 101 patients, and the rate at which physicians implemented pharmacist recommendations. Richmond Apothecaries received very encouraging results, documenting that pharmacists' interventions could result in glucose levels being decreased significantly and that a 90% medication adherence rate could be achieved and maintained. Physicians eventually implemented 75% of pharmacist recommendations.

In addition to developing optimal collaborative practice approaches with physicians, other areas are also being developed. Currently, obtaining provider numbers, billing third parties for service, and producing standards of quality for their pharmaceutical care process are their priorities.

> You make a living by what you get, but you make a life by what you give.
>
> —Winston Churchill

"We don't charge patients for routine programs, although we have demonstrated how these services are different from what they may have experienced previously, and most would be willing to pay," notes Herbert. "We don't want to lose patients over a few dollars for services and we would rather concentrate on payment from third parties." Shibley says that this is a key priority for her right now and they intend to work diligently and persistently until efforts pay off. Herbert says, "The dollars are not the motivator to providing good patient care; they are the by-product. Professionals have to do their best for the patients they serve." He sees this as one of the greatest challenges of widely implementing pharmaceutical care and believes that the formation of performance-based networks with third-party payers will be needed before pharmaceutical care can become mainstream within pharmacy.

No great enterprise will ever begin if all obstacles must first be overcome.

—Napoleon Hill

Shibley is working on standards of quality outputs from pharmaceutical care services so that physicians, patients, and others know what to expect. "Right now, there is no set process that is widely accepted as the optimal, integrated system for collaboration with physicians. To further implement and build acceptance of pharmaceutical care by others, I think this [process] is needed."

Herbert, Shibley, and the other Richmond Apothecaries staff continue to share their experiences generously and view networking activities as one key to their success. "No matter where an idea starts or goes, I learn something every time I attend a professional program," says Shibley. She recently had the opportunity to learn from 50 colleagues at the APhA Foundation's Advanced Practice Institute in Florida. Herbert shares Shibley's enthusiasm for networking, believing, "No matter what you know, you can always learn. While we served as expert faculty for the Project ImPACT: Hyperlipidemia Program, we picked up many good ideas from its participants. We are pleased to be part of APhA Foundation's new Asthma Quality Improvement Pilot."

Besides her father's influence, Michelle Shibley credits several college professors for her professionalism. She is quick to thank Tom Reinders, Pharm.D., and Jim McKenny, Pharm.D., at the Medical College of Virginia; and Dennis Clifton, Pharm.D., and Chris Isreal, Pharm.D., at the University of Kentucky. She met Dr. Clifton and Dr. Isreal during her post-graduate residency program. She credits Joanne Holly, Pharm.D., for encouraging her to enroll in the program. Shibley will also tell you that as a young student she resisted being a pharmacist because she wanted to "do her own thing," but when it came right down to a decision, she enjoyed the interaction with people so much that she knew pharmacy was right for her. "Besides," she says, "I once spent a summer working in an [ice cream] restaurant and that taught me [that] such work is not [my] life's goal."

How does this busy mother of two find balance in her life? "I run and recently completed a half marathon, and I find time to paint in watercolors," she says. "But when I get a full day off, I like to play with my kids, go to the beach or enjoy the pleasures of gardening." It used to be hard for Shibley to leave work behind, but with two children she says she would not have enough energy to devote to family if she took her job home with her. "I find my involvement with my family is re-energizing and refreshing. Finally, my faith and religion are very important to me, so I volunteer to work in our church health ministry."

There is no real excellence in all this world which can be separated from right living.

—Davis Starr Jordan

When asked to describe herself, Shibley uses words like "creative intelligence" and "high integrity." "I think my integrity is the most important aspect of my professional demeanor," she says "it is the source of what makes my success solid and sustainable. Having creative intelligence means I have the street smarts to apply myself and persevere. If I were to be remembered by my patients, I think they would see me as a pharmacist who took a personal interest in their health and cared about how they were doing. Further, if I were to be remembered by my pharmacy colleagues, it would be as someone who is self-directed and determined to persevere."

Asked if she reads any books in the management or communications field for inspiration, Shibley cites authors such as Stephen R. Covey, Wayne Dyer, and Deepak Chopra. A book she recently read and liked is *Who Moved My Cheese* by Stephen Johnson, M.D. "A fascinating figure that I admire and like to read about is Jacqueline Onassis," she adds. "Here was an independent woman who did her own thing despite the odds and tragedy in her life."

We could never learn to be brave and patient if there were only joy in the world.

—Helen Keller

One important lesson for Schibley did not come from a book or from a mentor; it occurred when she was asked to do some teaching. "I found a student who I thought did not care to learn, yet expected a higher grade," she relates, "and this taught me not to put my expectations onto others. I may be hard on myself, and yet I learned through that experience I cannot expect the same performance from others."

ADVICE TO OTHERS

Michelle Shibley offers these words of wisdom for others to follow:

- Be diligent and persistent, as it is being determined that gets you there. It will bring rewards. Change takes time.
- Be willing to share your successes and lessons learned with others, and listen to their experiences. It is one of the best sources of encouragement and new ideas.
- Have fun! We love what we do every day and would never return to the way we practiced before.
- Be optimistic, look forward and believe in what you do.
- On the payment challenge, stay positive. As one of her father's mentors once told her, "You will never be paid more for what you do until you do more than what you're paid to do."
- Success comes when one gets the following into balance and sync —professional work, home life, and your faith journey.
- Always remember that traffic moves in many directions, there is always a route for you that will take you where you want to go.

16

KIM SWIGER: TEACHER AND MOTIVATOR

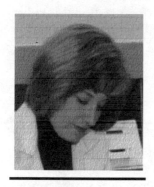

Kim Swiger

When Kim Malone Swiger graduated from the Medical College of Virginia (MCV)'s School of Pharmacy in the mid-1980s her career goal was to "interact and build relationships with patients." She says, "I had worked for a community pharmacist in high school and it really reinforced my decision to become a pharmacist. I knew I liked the health care field, but found many of the tasks performed in a doctor's office by the nursing staff unappealing." The profession is lucky to have Swiger. She sets an example as a teacher and motivator to patients and colleagues alike.

Swiger did not expect that her efforts would place her in a small but growing group of leading-edge practitioners who are all devoted to helping patients receive the intended benefit of their medications through pharmaceutical care practice. In fact, she does not see herself as an innovator or visionary at all. Rather, she sees herself as "a doer" who is motivated to implement better patient care.

It is by acts and not by ideas that people live.

—Anatole France

The actions of men are the best interpreters of their thoughts.

—John Locke

The thing she likes most about her work is the teaching aspect — whether a patient or colleague. "I find it rewarding to watch people develop." She has had a number of opportunities to do so as the manager of pharmacy operations for Ukrop's Supermarket Pharmacies in Richmond, VA. She credits a number of her own teachers with creating the vision she has been able to execute. Among these mentors and models is John Beckner, Ukrop's director of pharmacy and whole health, a true innovator who has been widely recognized for his leadership, most recently with the Jacob W. Miller Award from the APhA Foundation. Another teacher she credits for influencing her is MCV's Ralph Small. "He was a big advocate for organizational involvement and I got to know him through work with the Virginia Pharmacists' Association (VPhA). He was instrumental in our decision to apply to, and eventually participate in, the APhA Foundation's Project ImPACT: Hyperlipidemia Program," she notes.

It was there she met a teacher of whom she speaks highly, Ben Bluml, the APhA Foundation's vice president of research who directs Project ImPACT programs. "Ben is very motivating. He works with many practitioners around the country and shares stories among project participants regarding their challenges and successes with patients," Swiger says. She considers her participation in Project ImPACT among the big turning points in her life, solidifying her goals to implement patient care.

MERGING PERSONAL AND COMPANY GOALS

"I think it is critical for you to like and enjoy your job, because there will be challenges along the way implementing services," Swiger advises. That said, Ukrop's continues to be involved in an expanding array of patient-care programs that build on the corporation's mission statement (Figure 16.1).

It is part of the company's larger vision, mission, and shared values to be a world-class provider of food and services.

Those values are readily apparent in the chain. Ukrop's is an innovative, high-volume company whose pharmacies are located in primarily upper-middle-class suburbs of Richmond. Its phamacists fill 1300 to 1600 prescriptions per week. The 27-store chain has 19 pharmacies, 15 of which offer wellness centers. Ukrop's is a family-owned

We believe food and pharmacy go together and that our stores provide a natural setting for pharmacy departments. Our goal is to help our customers live healthier, happier, and longer lives by providing them a wide assortment of products and services designed to foster wellness. We believe our pharmacy commitment of "Taking Care of People" is a natural extension of our ongoing commitment to being "Where People and Food Come First."

The mission of Ukrop's is to serve our customers and community efficiently and effectively while treating our customers, associates, and suppliers as we personally like to be treated. We will achieve profitable growth and long-term financial success while promoting an atmosphere of mutual trust, honesty, and integrity.

We believe we can best fulfill our vision and accomplish our mission by living these values daily:

- Superior customer service — resulting from great execution, a caring attitude, and a sense of urgency
- Honesty and fairness — acting openly, equitably, and consistently in all we do
- Superior quality and freshness — uncompromising in our commitment
- Cost consciousness — minimizing waste and vigorously pursuing continuous improvement, resulting in lower prices and greater values
- Teamwork — coming together as a diverse workforce to achieve our shared vision
- Atmosphere — fostering an environment that is safe, clean, challenging, and fun
- Health and fitness — strengthening our bodies for productive and creative minds
- Competence — performing our jobs effectively and being informed and excited about our food and services
- Lifelong learning — seeking knowledge and enthusiastically sharing it with others
- Quality of life — committing to improving the lives of our families and well-being of our community

Figure 16.1   Ukrop's Mission Statement

business with a team-oriented, customer service culture. Its strategy is to set itself apart from more traditional chain pharmacies by focusing on healthy lifestyles.

The company has a number of innovative programs and services, including food and healthy eating resources, health screenings for blood glucose, cholesterol, blood pressure, mammography, and the Shape-Up exercise plan. Smoking cessation, diabetes, hypertension, and asthma pharmaceutical care services are provided. The pharmacies are active with Project ImPACT: Osteoporosis, a pharmaceutical care service and payment demonstration model that identifies patients at mid-to-high risk for the condition. The staff refers patients to physicians for treatment, and payment for the service comes from HealthSouth Corporation, a large managed-care provider in the area.

CHANGING VISION

"My vision of the type of relationship I [want to] build with patients has changed tremendously during the last few years that I have been active in pharmaceutical care. You become a source of information that you couldn't expect when starting early in your career." During her first 5 years of practice with another busy pharmacy chain, Swiger was able to build personal relationships with patients, but the focus was on earning confidence, trust, and ensuring that patients understand the medications they were taking. Now, she builds on the foundation of confidence and trust to help patients with diet, nutrition, disease management, and therapy monitoring. "It is helping them with much greater detail," she says.

EARNEST BEGINNINGS

Her work in pharmaceutical care began in 1996, when she and five other pharmacist colleagues participated in a MedOutcomes disease state management training program. "John Beckner was able to build on the company's strong health focus and customer service by expanding that thinking into the pharmacy. The senior executives understood that pharmacy was changing and they needed to make a long-term investment in building the pharmaceutical care business. Formal disease state management training was the first step."

Other training programs they have availed themselves of during the intervening years include APhA and VPhA offerings in immunization and hyperlipidemia. They have participated in the APhA Foundation's Advanced Practice Institutes and, more recently, the University of Tennessee's diabetes training program. Pharmacists at the company have been trained as well with a program developed in conjunction with MCV's Ralph Small for in-house use.

Swiger keeps up on her knowledge base by participating in local, state, and national programs as well as reading on her own. "We are a training site for MCV Pharm.D. candidates. They are a another great source of continuing education. During our monthly pharmacy meetings, the students will present in-services to us. Our partnership with the school has also provided us with the opportunity to learn from community pharmacy residents and professors. For example, assistant professor Kelly Gude helped us to receive our CLIA certification to be able to do cholesterol and blood glucose screenings."

SERVICES BLOOM

After the initial MedOutcomes training, pharmacies began offering services that included instruction in how to manage asthma, diabetes, hypertension, and hyperlipidemia. The pharmacy also had a disease state management contract with a local HMO for patients with asthma and diabetes. Since then, the diabetes program has been expanded to include a comprehensive set of services, including a seven-class education program, hemoglobin A1C monitoring, and care offered at four locations.

At first, however, making the practice succeed took a lot of personal capital and commitment. Often the staff arrived before work and on Saturdays to schedule and meet with patients. "While each wellness center pharmacy had monthly screening, many patients required regular follow-up and we found appointments to be very effective. You have to really want this type of practice to succeed and be willing to do what it takes. The rewards are worth it." The wellness center staff has since moved away from scheduling appointments for service, because the scheduling was difficult to sustain and manage. Building service today is more focused on identifying patients through screenings. Over 160 are offered at 13 locations with up to 900 people participating.

MARKETING SERVICES

Marketing services to internal staff, patients, and physicians has been key. Explaining the new services to staff was an important start. "We needed to help store managers, employees, and pharmacy technicians understand how the services could help patients and the company." An interesting example is the requests Swiger often received from store personnel to use the space in the wellness center for other reasons. "Maximizing floor space is a goal for any chain operation. It is hard for people accustomed to working toward that goal to see some space not necessarily being used all the time. I was very flexible and it became a nonissue in short order."

A variety of ways to reach people who may be candidates for pharmaceutical care services have been instituted. In the monthly customer newsletter, *Great News*, a piece that focuses on nutrition and health has been helpful. Screenings are advertised in newspaper ads. In addition to direct marketing through newsletters and letters to patients, 2-week screening schedules are posted in the stores.

Physician marketing can be a challenge. The staff has learned that long-term relationship building is effective and has developed important connections with the Richmond Academy of Medicine. When the team undertakes new programs, such as Project ImPACT: Osteoporosis, it works to educate the physician community in advance and thereby helps build awareness of the positive results such programs can produce. They have also invited several family practitioners to tour the pharmacy and see the services offered first-hand.

PAYMENT FOR SERVICES

Ukrop's has a fee schedule for cholesterol, blood glucose, other screenings, in-depth counseling, and nutrition and diet consultations. Primarily, patients make payment, although Ukrop's is pursuing third-party payment, especially in light of its American Diabetes Association (ADA) certification. Additionally, Project ImPACT: Osteoporosis has a third-party payment demonstration component. Swiger reflects, "Patients understand the value and they receive a great benefit. It is fulfilling to see them get well."

Swiger hopes patients and colleagues will remember her for being caring, helpful in solving medication issues, hardworking, and willing to go the extra mile. "I think you should treat people the way you want your Mom or Dad to be treated," she says. That reflects some of the values she learned growing up in a blue-collar family with five siblings in the mid-size rural Maryland community of Salisbury. Early jobs common among young people included waiting tables at the local family-owned restaurant and in a bakery. She also volunteered in the local community pharmacy.

She has learned to embrace failure and cites two examples. The first was getting a B on a biology project — anything less than an A was not acceptable. But, her teacher said he did so because she needed to improve it before taking it to the local county science fair. She took his advice, earning a first prize ribbon in the event. She learned discipline from that experience, a trait she feels strongly contributed to where she is today.

The second life-changing experience was marrying and eventually divorcing her first husband. It was a difficult mistake and one she did not want to repeat. "It made me tougher, stronger," she reflects. "It made me appreciate life much more." That cheerful outlook attracted a neighbor, Brad, who later became her second husband and best friend.

Affairs of the heart are the most difficult mountains to climb in life.

—Alan Hobson

She also feels that getting along with people, loving one's profession, working hard, and persevering were critical components of her self-development.

They are traits she is learning to bring to her own growing family as well. She and her husband welcomed twins, Patrick and Caroline, into their lives this past year. It was the culmination of a long process addressing physical challenges to having children. "They are what I'm most proud of," Swiger beams. When she's not working hard helping others at Ukrop's, they like to go to the beach, stay at bed-and-breakfast inns, show their wire-haired fox terrier, or visit family. Prior to the twins' arrival, she and her husband had enjoyed a cooking tour of the Hudson Valley. She wishes she had more time for leisure reading these days, but managing the family comes first and is what she cares about most — that, and sharing with the twins some of the valuable life lessons she has learned.

ADVICE TO OTHERS

- Start small. Small things can make a huge difference. Everyone has a unique contribution to make; it requires taking time to "step outside the box" to see it.
- Be flexible. It happens one step at a time and requires personal commitment and capital, especially at the beginning.
- Take advantage of what others have learned. Networking with colleagues at Ukrop's at association meetings, training programs, and other events is a constant source of motivation and support. "It keeps the ball rolling," she says.

- Explain what you are doing and why to colleagues at your practice and other sites. To succeed, pharmaceutical care requires teamwork.
- Train technicians and store staff in their new roles. They will do a better job and help in marketing services when the opportunity arises over the phone or with customers. It also shows them you value them as team members.
- Partner with your local school of pharmacy. It is a win–win situation. They need to develop strong community pharmacy training sites and you can learn a tremendous amount from professors and students. Students are great — they challenge you to develop cases and other learning tools.
- Take every opportunity to participate in educational programs, whether they are local, state, or national. It reinforces what you are doing and expands your knowledge base.
- Step back occasionally and reevaluate the services you are offering. What is working? What is weak? What changes should you make to your goals and plans?

17

GREG WEDIN: DEFINING A PROCESS FOR PHARMACEUTICAL CARE

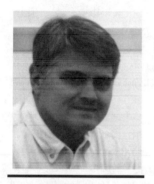

Greg Wedin

Long before today's books on pharmaceutical care were written, there were numerous practitioners who took on a great deal of risk to pursue their goal of providing patient care. They defined for others what that process of care looks like and how to apply it, whether comprehensively or among a select group of patients. Greg Wedin is one of them. This is his story. It is about being in the right place at the right time, and how, by following your vision and heart, obstacles can be overcome.

It's not whether you get knocked down. It's whether you get up again.

—Vince Lombardi

"It seems I've always wanted to do things that weren't the norm or widely accepted. As a result, I have always confronted resistance leading to either convincing or appeasing two crowds — those who need the service and those who want it too," Wedin reflects. He has spent almost 10 years creating, defining, and implementing pharmaceutical care programs himself, as well as supporting other pharmacists who do, and the time has been full of such challenges. Regarding his stoicism, you might believe the path was an easy one. But spend some time with Wedin and you begin to appreciate the many unsung heroes who laid the groundwork for countless other pharmacists who were willing to bear less risk to pursue patient care.

COMING HOME

Wedin's hometown of Glencoe, MN is a rural community of 4500 people, 50 miles west of the twin cities of Minneapolis and St. Paul. After nearly a decade away, Wedin returned in 1992 to work with his pharmacist father at their community's sole pharmacy, Wedin Drug. The lessons he learned while finding his own way proved to be the needed element for them to become part of a select group of 20 pharmacies that were part of the Minnesota Pharmaceutical Care Project. Pharmacist and pharmaceutical care theory co-creator Linda Strand, Ph.D., through the University of Minnesota College of Pharmacy's Peters Institute, directed the project. Its purpose was to bring Strand and fellow author Dr. Charles Hepler's defining 1990 paper on pharmacists solving drug therapy problems into actual practice. This project hoped to create the care process that today is often associated with thriving pharmaceutical care practices.

"I was literally in the pharmacy for only days when I learned they were recruiting pharmacists for the project," Wedin recalls. "I knew I wanted to do more than the traditional retail pharmacist — that is why I applied." The pharmacy was a traditional one, filling 80 to 100 prescriptions per day, with a heavy emphasis on cards and gifts and a large front-end as part of its 4000 sq. ft. After being selected to be part of the program, the Wedins remodeled the store to build a workflow and counseling area.

THE MINNESOTA PROJECT

The project entailed providing comprehensive services to a group of BC/BS patients. The work entailed identifying whether any of the eight categories of drug-related problems, outlined by Strand and Hepler, applied to a patient and creating a plan to resolve them.

"It was not an easy thing to implement. My 'ah ha' moment finally came when I visited fellow project pharmacist, John Loch (also one of the 16 pharmacists featured in the APhA/NWDA Concept Pharmacy Project). He was [dispensing] more prescriptions than we were but there was less commotion and it looked a lot smoother. That led me to go back to the pharmacy and institute a few workflow changes. First, we separated the prescription entry and pick-up areas and staffed the entry with pharmacists who could interview the patients and get needed information in one step. The actual prescription-filling process was done by a pharmacy technician with the pharmacist providing the final check, managing the DUR process, and delivering the prescriptions to the patients," Wedin remembers.

For all new prescriptions, their safety, effectiveness, and indications were assessed and patients were followed up at 3-month intervals. Appointments are always made for the first-time patient to the pharmacy. A paper-based system for documenting care was used. At that time, turnkey pharmaceutical care software programs did not exist and feedback was not provided to the patient's physician or other caregivers. "You have to [remember] that this project was about defining the process of care. It was trial and error and even the pharmacists who participated did not always have a clear understanding of how we would do it," says Wedin.

With regard to the physicians, no formal meetings were held, but Wedin believes the small town practice environment would have supported such an idea. "It would have been valuable in hindsight," he notes. While there were no problems experienced, it could have helped "legitimize" the practice in his point of view and help define the pharmacist's relationship with the physician in providing collaborative care.

Another regret was the lack of staff education. "We did not educate the staff or get their buy-in on the project. They knew what we were doing was different but they were not sure why. It would have been more helpful to have done this, especially with the front-end staff."

BC/BS paid for the patient services and pharmacies were not allowed to charge patients directly. Many patients were not aware of the payment system. Payments were made using a RBRVS at a rate of about $7 per intervention or $60 per hour. Wedin was monitoring several hundred patients during the course of the 3-year pilot and the pharmacy was one of ten that completed the whole program when it ended in 1995.

ROLE OF EXPERIENCE AND TRAINING

"My Pharm.D. helped but I don't think it was necessary for participation. I do think there is a lot that needs to be done to help pharmacists understand their role but I don't think training/credentialing is always necessary," he reflects. Wedin drew more from his experiences with poison control centers and toxicology for the clinical knowledge used in the care process. A vision he repeats several times during the interview is that providing pharmaceutical care is no different from what many pharmacists do whenever a family member or friend asks for their advice. "Just because it is being applied to a patient in the pharmacy, it is not different. You are answering questions, identifying and resolving problems with therapy, and making sure it is right." he notes.

Even though his prior practical experience was clinical, the project still represented a turning point for Wedin. "I really came to understand what [my] purpose as a pharmacist was in terms of identifying and solving drug-related problems." Another turning point occurred during a retreat at pharmacy school when a fellow student became ill and Wedin came to his aid. A clinical professor, who had observed his actions, encouraged him to pursue practice beyond dispensing.

He decided to pursue his Pharm.D. degree, one of ten students in a highly respected and competitive program. He pursued nontraditional rotations and took a fellowship at the University of Maryland's Poison Control Center in 1983. The Hennepin County Poison Control Center director, Ed Krenzlok, was a big influence on Wedin, as was the program's outgoing fellow who said the experience had been the best of his life. Wedin was convinced and moved East. "I knew I would do something other than work in Wedin Drug. First, the store could not support two of us. Second, my Dad felt I would never earn credibility with the community unless I went away to work for a while."

His father was a huge influence on his pursuing a pharmacy career, unlike his two brothers and two sisters who pursued business management, vocational/technical, and medical technology fields. "I saw how people in the community respected my father and valued the help he provided. It was an honorable profession that could provide a comfortable life and a good career path with many options," he says.

When the time with mentor Gary Dirda at the University of Maryland was ending, Wedin learned of a position being created in West Virginia for a poison control center director with a joint appointment on the faculty at the school of pharmacy. He worked relief until the position materialized and moved to Charleston in 1984. It proved to be an important learning experience.

LESSONS LEARNED IN PRACTICE

"While I don't consider myself having had any real failures," says Wedin, "there were battles and I took heat for my aggressive approach to fulfilling my goal to make the poison center recognized regionally within the shortest time frame possible." It was a challenge upon his arrival, when he learned that the staff was poorly trained, protocols had not been established, and resources were few. "I was young and energetic and had an 'I'm going to do it' kind of attitude," he notes.

Another interesting coincidence was that he arrived at the new position one month after the chemical plant tragedy in Bopal, India, involving methylisocyanate. The only other factory in the world using that toxic substance was a mere 20 miles away from Charleston.

Difficulties strengthen the mind, as labor does the body.

—Seneca

His work in the next 8 years involved service, teaching, and research and Wedin was given tenure as an associate professor. The time in West Virginia also gave him the chance to meet and marry his wife Susan, who was from the Charleston area and lived in the same apartment complex. They dated and "hung out at the pool" for 4 years before becoming engaged and marrying. They have two daughters, ages 4 and 8. "Susan is a strong person and I really appreciated her support of our relocation back to Minnesota in 1992." Wedin had begun to witness resources declining at the poison control center, and if this continued he could foresee the potential recurrence of the same problems he had previously solved. He did not want to turn the center around a second time. So he gave 6 months notice, and recruited and trained his replacement.

MOVING AS COINCIDENCE

As it turns out, in spite of moving away from one family to another, the Minnesota decision proved important in another significant way. In 1998, Susan was diagnosed with chronic myelogenous leukemia, requiring intensive chemotherapy, bone marrow transplant, and follow-up care. "Had we stayed in West Virginia, we would have had to move and live near the closest treatment center." In Minnesota, the University of Minnesota was only an hour away, allowing the Wedins to stay in their Glencoe home, draw on their circle of friends, family, and church for support during the long treatments.

In prosperity our friends know us; in adversity we know our friends.

—John Churton Collins

"In my life, I am most proud of my wife and the way she battled her way back from cancer. She used her strength and faith to recover. She uses it every day to raise our children and manage our home, especially with me being away so much," reflects Greg. "The experience expanded my faith as well. Susan had come from a strong background in the Nazarene faith. I am much more involved now. Her bout with cancer also was a turning point in my career. As a pharmacist, while you understand the science of disease, this put a face on it for me at a fundamental level. It showed us what is important and changed how we live on a day-to-day basis."

And that is reflected in what Wedin does when he is home and off work. They enjoy each other's company as a family by watching movies, listening to music, and accomplishing simple things around the house. Disney World was a popular vacation spot but home works just fine too. Occasionally when he is on the road, Wedin enjoys a round of golf as well. "Our vacations are really pretty subdued and simple," he notes

A man should always consider how much he has more than he wants, and how much more unhappy he might be than he really is.

—Joseph Addison

HELPING OTHERS SEE THE LIGHT

So where did his experience as a pharmaceutical care innovator lead him? Wedin is now the director of professional services for AmerisourceBergen and is responsible for creating programs that support pharmacist patient-care activities and working with manufacturers as well. The position grew out of the Minnesota project when it ended in 1995. Participants realized there was a need to continue to implement pharmaceutical care and the university did not have the ability to train large numbers of pharmacists. A private sector solution was sought; Amerisource became involved early on.

Wedin had expressed interest in training pharmacists and was hired to do that on a contract basis. He worked at Wedin Drug for 4 days each week and provided training through Pharmaceutical Care Minnesota Group in his remaining time. A 3-day comprehensive training program was created, and as things evolved his job became full time.

He has learned a lot in the intervening 6 years, going from a practitioner/creator of the care process to a teacher/trainer of others to a promoter of whatever it takes to support a pharmacist who wants to move forward. "First, we discovered the system in general was not ready for a large number of pharmacists to be practicing comprehensive pharmaceutical care. It was more than many could conceptualize or adopt. Those willing to take the risk did so. Others were not willing."

"Second, we learned that you had to be dedicated to it. You had to believe this is what you needed to be doing as a pharmacist and be willing to expend resources with no guaranteed payback. Some people could conceptually embrace the practice, but not internalize it."

"Third, we learned it is a very individual decision. There are a significant number of pharmacists who have implemented patient care without a lot of support from groups. They are entrepreneurs at heart."

He believes that for pharmacists to be ultimately fulfilled, they need to embrace their patient care role. "You can convince some practitioners to move ahead. But, here at AmerisourceBergen, we have repositioned ourselves instead to support whatever activities pharmacists want to do vs. convincing them to do something else or do it differently." A good example is their health-screening program that provides support whether a pharmacist wants to counsel and conduct the screening, counsel only, or delegate it to other screening personnel.

He also believes that comprehensive pharmaceutical care is a vision for which to work hard, but it will not happen on a widespread scale until the system infrastructure supports it. Until then, many practitioners are approaching patient care in a focused fashion based on certain diseases. "And, that is okay," he says, "as long as pharmacists are doing something that puts [them] in direct contact with the patient. Because when they do come face to face with them, patients learn they have easy access to knowledgeable people who can answer their questions and solve their problems. It provides reinforcement to patients and they begin to demand the services."

He hopes to remain part of the profession's transition for many years to come. "I can see myself [being] happy doing similar things as [I am] today [which] support where pharmacy needs to go. I think I'll continue to work incrementally toward the vision of comprehensive pharmaceutical care and hope, in 20 years, we [will] have the systems and structures in place to make it common." His former patients in Glencoe already know he has made a difference and they tell him how much they miss the care they received after Wedin Drug closed a few years back. "They know we cared about them as people and their health. At the end of the day, that's what gets me excited — meeting people's needs."

ADVICE TO OTHERS

- Put yourself face to face with patients. It is a good place to start. You'll find yourself doing more because the patients will demand it.
- Delegate what tasks you can to others, focus on the patients.
- Be disciplined, work hard, and persevere.
- Learn the ability to take and manage risk.
- Mental toughness can help you through obstacles. Build it up.

III

LESSONS LEARNED
FROM PASSIONATE
PHARMACISTS

18

WHERE DO YOU GO FROM HERE?

Believe in the impossible, hold tight to the incredible, and live each day
to its fullest potential. You can make a difference in your world.

—Rebecca Barlow Jordan

Pharmacist trailblazers seem to share common attributes and provide
similar advice to those who share their desire to help move comprehensive pharmacist-provided patient care forward. Those whom we
interviewed are trailblazers and innovators and they all tend to follow
a pattern that Everett Rogers described in his book, *Diffusion of
Innovation*, wherein he states:

- It takes time for people to innovate, but the overall pattern is
  predictable.
- The pattern of an adoption process can be seen in distinct
  phases.
- It is possible to apply different characteristics to identify those
  who innovate, dependent upon how quickly they accept and
  implement their innovation.

Everett Rodgers describes his pattern of innovation as a seven-step
sequence:

- Developing the need for change
- Establishing an information-exchange relationship with
  stakeholders

- Diagnosing the problems of clients
- Creating an intent to change clients
- Translating the intent into action
- Stabilizing adoption and preventing discontinuances
- Moving the client toward a degree of self-sufficiency

While the people featured in this book had different personal pathways to creating new practice paradigms, they have one thing in common. They were zealous in their quest to initiate a new practice model that moved from just dispensing a product to one that included helping people. Or, to put it more succinctly, as Curt Barr says, "It was a matter of leaving the pharmaceutical model behind and adapting the medical care model. I believed that people take drugs and my responsibility only began with dispensing drugs and did not stop once I had those drugs in little bottles."

All of our interviewees realized nothing would change the profession they loved unless they took responsible action. They counted on an inner voice that drove them forward and, in several cases, to near failure, but they kept trying until they saw progress.

The lessons these special pharmacists shared about their successes and challenges carry important insights. We assembled the lessons learned in our conversations with them into the following checklist. It is quite possible you may say, "Yes, yes, that's me," after you compare yourself with this checklist.

A PHARMACEUTICAL CARE CHECKLIST: 14 QUESTIONS TO ASSESS IF YOU HAVE WHAT IT TAKES

1. Do you have a passion for patients and the profession?

Among our interviewees, there was a 100% commitment on their part to the profession of pharmacy and the patients they serve. Each pharmacist carried a strong desire to help people and make good on the covenant of all professionals. Our interviewees were able to ask themselves every day when they went to work, "Why am I here today?" To them the answer was easy, "I am here to make a difference."

All success consists in this: You are doing something for somebody —
benefiting humanity — and the feeling of success comes from the consciousness of this.

—Elbert Hubbard

Joy is not in things, it is in us.

—Richard Wagner

2. Do you know who you are and do you have a support system in place?

Just as our interviewees were boldly selecting career paths in community-based pharmaceutical care, they also had personal and professional support in the form of wives, husbands, family, friends, and
mentors. Such support was the basis of their self-confidence and
renewal of energy. Their support systems were also used to test ideas
and were stronger influences than professional societies. Although
continuing professional education in a variety of areas was commonplace, these pharmacists shared a strong need to keep up and to learn
where the opportunities are. To them networking was a way to obtain
stimulation and discuss new ideas.

3. Can you tell others what you are doing?

It was important for our interviewees to have a written mission statement and a goals statement and to communicate this, in lay language,
to fellow staff, all patients, and all providers that come into view. As
Laurie Kaup pointed out, "Our mission is to take care of patients as
if they are family," and she never forgets it. Technicians and all store
staff need to be trained in the new paradigm because if it is ever going
to succeed in a community setting it will require teamwork.

The important thing is this: to be able at any moment to sacrifice what
we are for what we could become.

—Charles du Bois

4. Do you have the courage to act?

Turning your vision of professional growth and opportunity into a reality is a difficult thing to do. But our interviewees believed the only way they could grow professionally and have the satisfaction of helping others was to walk a trail forged by their own ideas. They had given great thought to their role as pharmacists and the greater role of the profession within society and so moved ahead believing they were doing the right thing. Our interviewees saw their journey on the trail of pharmaceutical care as a journey and not a destination. They found it to be a trail made up of many large and small adventures. They also knew it involved taking a risk that likely could transform them into professionals that were different, but they went ahead anyway. Our interviewees were very willing to ask themselves as they embarked on another step to reach their goal, "what is the worst thing that can happen."

Clear your mind of can't.

—Samuel Johnson

The road to success leads through the valley of humility, and the path is up the ladder of patience and across the wide barren plains of perseverance. As yet, no short cut has been discovered.

—Joseph Lamb

5. Have you been able to learn from your mistakes?

While our interviewees reported little in the way of failure, those who did saw failure as a learning experience and moved on. Keep in mind what one interviewee told us, "Sometimes when you reach a roadblock you just have to put things on the back-burner until society catches up." The key here is if you think you are wrong, move on from where you are. Success comes from pushing the limits of your experience and finding new ways to think about what you may have left behind.

6. Do you enjoy a balanced lifestyle?

The "dare to be different" pharmacists we interviewed put a lot of time and effort into assuring themselves and their families that their life was in balance, i.e., emotionally, physically, and spiritually. While they put in long hours building their unique pharmaceutical care practices their spiritual and family lives were very important to them and thus they were committed to being physically fit and using vacations, hobbies, sports, and other activities to keep their lives in perspective. They knew how important immediate family members were in their lives and the need to nurture those relationships.

> Things which matter most should never be at the expense of things that matter the least.
>
> —Goethe

7. Have you stopped learning?

Our interviewees were never afraid to put themselves in new and challenging situations for they knew that was how they would grow. To them networking was a huge and positive support to learn from others without reinventing the wheel. State, local, county, and national professional societies were all good places to continue learning.

8. Are you developing professional partnerships with colleges of pharmacy?

We found many innovative pharmacists partnering with their schools and colleges of pharmacy. They found this was not only a source of the latest clinical and professional trends, but an opportunity for them to formalize their innovative practices by trying to teach their ways to others. Since all schools and colleges need community training sites, there is much to be learned by their faculty and students, especially when a concept like pharmaceutical care has no strong parameters and can become the basis of case studies with many variations.

9. Are you willing to start small?

Our interviewees all started in a small way and made it grow. To them pharmaceutical care did not become an overnight sensation. Since small things can grow into huge differences, it took time for each of our innovators to think and step outside their traditional pharmacy "box" and stepwise to put processes and new programs in place.

10. Do you see the glass as half empty or half full?

Our interviewees were independent thinkers who saw opportunity and change as positive things. They had no self-doubts and surrounded themselves with positive role models. Too many people wait for the perfect time before they commit to anything. Such doubt has prevented many from moving forward and being active. Remember these words:

A good plan acted upon is better than a perfect plan that is never acted upon.

—General Eisenhower

11. Are you a good listener?

Pharmaceutical care requires that you respond to the patient's need. That means being a good listener so you "hear" what the patient's real concerns are. If you are not a good listener, take a course on active listening. It is an easily acquired skill and with a little practice can be mastered to open a whole new outlook on life.

12. Can you see pharmaceutical care as an investment?

If you are into pharmaceutical care because you want to make money, then you will need to spend money knowing it will take time before you find a return on that investment. Not every health plan, PBM, or TPA is willing to pay you just because you ask them to. You need investments in documentation systems and perhaps a remodeling of the physical site itself before you can walk the walk and talk the talk.

13. Are you involved in your community?

All the pharmacists that we interviewed were involved in church, social, and civic groups, and local, school, and professional societies. Being a part of the community became a great resource for knowing just how well their efforts were perceived. It is a truth that health care is like politics — it is all local.

14. Do you still believe in the values that make America great?

Our interviewees never wavered in their belief in the fundamental building blocks that define America as a country that rewards people who have integrity and work hard and persevere to reach a goal.

> Perseverance is a great element of success. If you only knock long enough and loud enough at the gate, you are sure to wake up somebody.
>
> —Henry Wadsworth Longfellow

The giant oak is an acorn that held its ground.

> —Anon.

At the start of the 21st century pharmacy is a rapidly changing world, one in which there is a shortage of pharmacists. In this era of uncertainty one of its challenges is to look to innovative practitioners and analytical thinkers to keep its members reflecting on the things that keep it prospering as a trusted helping profession.

As one of the learned professions, universities, professional societies, researchers from within and without, and public scrutinizers are clamoring to help. The question becomes: Are these people, most of whom have agendas that do not quite mesh with a public need, able to show the flexibility, openness, and diversity necessary to move a profession forward? The insights and experiences of these interviewees should become the essential dialogue for the profession. However, our concern is that they are having too much fun and finding too much success helping people and they will be missed from the leadership structures that purport to represent their profession.

We have enjoyed preparing this book for you and trust its insights succinctly sum up why some people have embraced the pharmaceutical care movement and found success doing it. We can assure you, based on our interviews, that helping people make the best use of their medications is a surefire way to rekindle your professional passion. We also believe the road to pharmaceutical care is not a destination, but a journey. As the new millennium unfolds there will be many traveling forward and raising the bar for new standards of practice to help an old, trusted, and honorable profession survive another millennium.

Finally, this piece of advice on success is shared by Curt Barr with each and every student with whom he comes into contact. It has stood the test of time and is the measure by which he tests whether or not he has been successful as a pharmacist.

I will be successful, says Curt Barr, when I am able:

To laugh often and much;
to win the respect of intelligent people
and the affection of children;
to earn the appreciation of honest critics
and endure the betrayal of false friends;
to appreciate beauty, to find the best in others;
to leave the world a bit better, whether by a healthy child,
a garden patch or a redeemed social condition;
to know even one life has breathed easier because you have lived.

—Ralph Waldo Emerson

Appendix

INTERVIEW GUIDE FOR PHARMACIST PROFILES

A: PRACTICE-BASED INFORMATION

- Tell me about the practice.
- How many sites?
- What type of neighborhood?
- What kinds of patients?
- How many prescriptions per day does the pharmacy dispense?
- How big is the pharmacy?
- How is it staffed? Number of technicians and pharmacists.
- Do you have any published articles on the practice you could send?
- How about pharmacy and personal photos?

B: PHARMACEUTICAL CARE SERVICES

- What pharmaceutical care services do you offer?
- Do you have a published mission or vision statement?
- Did you look at APhA or ASHP guidelines?
- Which services did you start with and why?
- How did you add on the other services?
- How quickly did you want to implement services and why?
- Did you look at any model or practice as a basis to begin yours?

C: MARKETING TO PATIENTS

- How do you enroll patients in your service programs?
- How do you market to patients?
- How do you get the word out that your practice offers these services?
- What marketing/selling messages have you used?
- What has worked and what hasn't?

D: PROCESS

- How many patients are you following in each area?
- How do you manage initial work-ups and follow-ups? Appointments?
- How long do the appointments take?
- Does it vary by disease or service offering?
- Do you offer any testing with the services (e.g., cholesterol, glucose, bone density)?

E: DOCUMENTATION

- How do you document the care provided?
- What information do you provide to patients and their physicians?
- Do you use software to document care or use some other method?
- Does it follow SOAP (subjective, objective, assessment, and plan) note format?
- Do you plan on getting software?
- When? How will you evaluate it?

F: MARKETING TO PHYSICIANS

- What have physicians' reactions been to your service offerings? How did you deal with them?
- How do you market to physicians?
- Have you ever invited physicians to an open house at the practice to see firsthand what you are doing?

G: MONEY MATTERS

- Do you bill patients or insurers for services?
- What billing forms do you use?
- What type of fee schedule do you use? How did you construct it?
- Have you looked at whether the payments cover costs? If so, how much?
- How much do you estimate you spent to get the services up and running (physical changes, education programs, etc.)?

H: WORKFLOW

- To implement services, what type of workflow changes did you make?
- Did you separate prescription inflow and pick-up areas?
- Do you have semiprivate or private counseling areas?
- Do you use automated voice mail systems? Fax systems? Other technology?

I: PERSONAL AND PERSONNEL TRAINING/NETWORKING/EDUCATION

- How did you get comfortable with your knowledge base within the areas you offer services?
- For what areas did your education prepare you? Did having a Pharm.D. or B.S. matter in your view?
- What training programs did you take? Who sponsored them?
- How did you educate the other pharmacy personnel? Other store personnel?
- How did you get corporate support? What were the greatest challenges/barriers?
- What role did networking play in your practice's development?

J: QUALITY IMPROVEMENT

- Have you evaluated services, how?
- Have you invited peers or patients in to provide feedback on the practice?

K: PERSONAL CHARACTERISTICS/LIFE EXPERIENCE

- Why/how did you get interested in pharmacy?
- Did you always know you wanted to be a patient-oriented pharmacist or did your goals change along the way?
- Are there people in your life, or in general, whom you particularly admire? Who and why?
- What can organizations do to support or stifle you?
- How did you come to be working here?
- How much time did it take between graduation and when you started? Was there a defining moment?
- What size town are you from and did you return? Are you living in a similar town?

L: PERSONAL DEVELOPMENT

- What is your vision for practice?
- What gets you excited?
- What has allowed you to become a better person?
- What skills did you acquire to be able to practice this way?
- What experiences were vital to your development?
- What were the turning points in your life?
- What role has failure played in your life? What did you learn from it?
- If you left your practice, what would you want your patients and colleagues to remember you for?
- If I called your colleagues and patients and asked what your strongest characteristics are, what would they say?
- What are you most proud of?
- What is the best decision you ever made in your life?
- What is your proudest moment?
- Can you name a management or communications guru?
- What is a good book you have recently read outside of the professional journals or magazines?
- Tell me about your family, brothers and sisters.
- Have there been one or two college professors that you admire or emulate?
- Who has provided advice that has helped in making your decision to practice differently?
- Have you sought advice from a mentor? Colleague? Family? Tax professional? Accountant? Lawyer? Corporate administrator?

- Is there someone special who gave you the courage to move ahead? Or did it come from within?
- What other associations or service providers were involved? If more than one, which was most helpful and why?
- What kind of hobbies do you have? How often are you able to engage in them?
- What do you do when you have a day off?
- Where do you take your vacations?
- How do you leave the office behind?
- What are your dreams?
- What do you stay up late at night thinking about?
- What are things you care about?
- How important is religion in your personal and professional life?
- How will you define success in your life?
- Since you have a choice to think positively or negatively about the world in which you live, how do you know when you will be successful?
- What do you do to keep from thinking negatively?
- What has been your biggest obstacle?
- If overcoming fear or worry is a key to your success, how do you do this?
- How did you develop a strong belief in yourself? Is it self-induced or does it come from someone? Is it faith-based?
- What are you doing, if anything, to reduce the risks associated with being self-employed?
- Have you studied the risk/profitability of providing pharmaceutical care before taking the plunge?
- Did you create a written business plan? Did you practice "due diligence?" Do you understand the growth and income potential?
- Is your decision based on more than financial success? Is it based on a desire to do something for society as a member of a helping profession?
- Choose from the following list those attributes you think are most responsible for your success:
    1. Discipline
    2. Getting along with people
    3. Loving one's profession
    4. Investing wisely in oneself
    5. Ability to inspire others as a team
    6. Working hard and persevering
    7. Ability to manage risk

8. Strong personal integrity
9. Focused on a professional niche
10. Regular exercise/sound body
11. Mental toughness? Sound mind?

■ Fear and panic are the result of an unconditioned mind/ body/spirit. Do you get fatigued? How do you manage work-related stress?

■ Which of the following labels would apply to you?
1. Innovator
2. Teacher
3. Professional
4. Motivator
5. Visionary
6. Other

■ Does "pharmaceutical care" enable you to fulfill all your professional hopes and dreams?

M: ADVICE TO OTHERS

■ If you could give several pointers to other people who want to build a pharmaceutical care practice, what would they be?

RECOMMENDED READING

The authors and interviewees recommend the following books as inspirational and informative texts that provide insight into the minds of those who dare to be different.

Bennis, W., *On Becoming a Leader*, Warren G. Bennis, Inc., Wilmington, MA, 1989, 226 pp.

Blanchard, K. and Bowles, S., *Gung Ho! Turn on the People in Any Organization*, William Morrow, New York, 1998, 184 pp.

Blanchard, K. and Bowles, S., *High Five: The Magic of Working Together*, HarperCollins, New York, 2001, 203 pp.

Canfield, J. et al., *Chicken Soup for the Soul at Work*, Health Communications, Inc., Deerfield Beach, FL, 1996, 330 pp.

Cook, J.R., *The Start-Up Entrepreneur*, Harper & Row, New York, 1986, 306 pp.

Covey, S.R., *The 7 Habits of Highly Effective People*, Simon & Schuster, New York, 1989, 358 pp.

Covey, S.R., *Living the 7 Habits*, Simon & Schuster, New York, 1999, 310 pp.

Douglas, M.R., *Making a Habit of Success*, Galahad Books, New York, 1999, 441 pp.

Fulghum, R. *All I Really Need to Know I Learned in Kindergarten*, Villard Books, New York, 1988, 196 pp.

Hobson, A., *From Everest to Enlightenment: An Adventure of the Soul*, Inner Everests, Inc., Calgary, Canada, 1999, 323 pp.

Johnson, S. and Blanchard, K.H., *Who Moved My Cheese? An Amazing Way to Deal with Change in Your Work and in Your Life*, Putnam, New York, 1998, 94 pp.

Jouzes, J. and Pozner, B., *Credibility*, Jossey-Bass, San Francisco, 1993, 332 pp.

Lustbader, W., *What's Worth Knowing?* Jeremy P. Tarcher/Putnam, New York, 2001, 243 pp.

Redfield, J., *The Celestine Prophecy*, Warner Books, New York, 1993, 246 pp.

Redfield, J., *The Tenth Insight,* Warner Books, New York, 1996, 236 pp.

Steele, J., Hiles, C., and Coburn, J., *Breakthrough to Peak Performance*, Catalyst Group, London, 1999, 266 pp.

Tannen, D., *You Just Don't Understand: Women and Men in Conversation*, Ballantine Books, New York, 1990, 330 pp.

Ventrella, S.W., *The Power of Positive Thinking: Ten Traits for Maximum Results*, Free Press, New York, 2001, 178 pp.

INDEX